A TEXTBOOK OF
MEDICAL CONDITIONS FOR
PHYSIOTHERAPISTS

by the same author

PHYSIOTHERAPY IN SOME SURGICAL CONDITIONS

A TEXTBOOK OF
MEDICAL CONDITIONS FOR
PHYSIOTHERAPISTS

BY

JOAN E. CASH

B.A., F.C.S.P, Dip. T.P.

Revised edition with additional chapters
by specialist contributors

FABER & FABER LIMITED

3 Queen Square

London

First published in 1951
by Faber & Faber Limited
3 Queen Square London W.C.1
Reprinted 1951 and 1954
Second edition 1957
Reprinted 1959 and 1962
Third edition 1965
Reprinted 1968
Fourth edition 1971
Reprinted 1973
Printed in Great Britain by
Alden & Mowbray Ltd
at the Alden Press, Oxford

ISBN 0 571 04733 5

Foreword

F. D. HOWITT

C.V.O., M.A., M.D., F.R.C.P.

Physician, with charge of Physical Medicine, Middlesex Hospital
Honorary Consultant in Physical Medicine to the Army
Senior Physician to the Arthur Stanley Institute for Rheumatic Diseases

IT GIVES ME PARTICULAR PLEASURE to write a short foreword to this book, partly because I have read it with great interest, and partly because I am convinced that it supplies a long-felt need.

The face of medicine in this country has changed considerably in recent years, mainly as the result of dire necessity imposed upon us by two World Wars. It has become less departmentalised, and has assumed a more purposeful character. We have come to realise that the achievement and maintenance of health, the conduct of serious disease and injury, and the rehabilitation and revocation of disabled persons are, none of them, a one-man job. Success can only be achieved by team-work, and in this team there are no two members more important than the doctor and the physiotherapist. Each has his separate function to fulfil, yet neither can fulfil it adequately unless he works in harmony with the other.

I suspect that Miss Cash had some difficulty in selecting the title for her book. It would manifestly be an impertinence for a doctor to write a textbook on physiotherapy for doctors, although there is great need for such a work. For it is most important that before prescribing the various forms of physical treatment, a medical man should be fully conversant with their uses and abuses, actions and reactions, indications and contra-indications. He should also realise the difficulties which beset the physiotherapist, when faced with an incorrect or inadequate prescription. It would be equally presumptuous for a physiotherapist to attempt to write a textbook on medicine for physiotherapists. Yet it is vital that the physiotherapist should appreciate the problems which the doctor has to face when assessing the likely value of physiotherapy in conjunction with other medical measures; its effect upon the constitutional and psychological condition of the patient;

its prospects and sometimes its dangers. All physical treatments, whether preventive, corrective or remedial should be welded into a general and organised scheme. These are the points which Miss Cash has so admirably stressed from the viewpoint of the physiotherapist.

The author has aimed at simplicity, both in the general lay-out and in the description of the various medical conditions. The rationale for treatment has been fully explained in each instance, and there is a refreshing freedom from extravagant claims. It is up to date, and should serve equally as a work of reference for the qualified physiotherapist and for the senior student preparing for her diploma.

FRANK HOWITT

Preface to the First Edition

IN WRITING THIS BOOK the author has not attempted to teach any new material but rather to explain in detail some of the medical conditions most often seen in a department of physical medicine. It is, therefore, a book for students of physiotherapy, and it is hoped that with a better understanding of the changes occurring in these conditions the physical treatment may be carried out with a greater degree of intelligence, interest and improved efficiency.

The subject matter covers many medical conditions, but it was felt that a chapter on physical treatment in the surgical group of respiratory conditions should be included, as many chest conditions alternate between surgical and medical treatment and the physiotherapist is required to treat cases throughout both stages.

Each chapter, as well as describing medical conditions, is followed by a short outline dealing with the broad principles of treatment of these conditions by physical measures. In certain of these diseases there is little information available about the physical treatment, and so to fill in this gap a fuller account has been given.

Preface to the Third Edition

MANY PHYSIOTHERAPISTS have contributed to this new edition of Miss Cash's much-read textbook and Mrs. Rosemary Smith has helped to gather together this team. With modern advances in all branches of medicine, physiotherapy has become more and more specialised and a number of experts have contributed chapters on their specialities in this edition.

Preface to the Fourth Edition

For this fourth edition, the author and her collaborators have made additions and alterations throughout the book. There is a new section on neoplasia and on acute infective polyneuritis. New matter on cervical spondylosis has been added and a new chapter on disseminated sclerosis, the Parkinsonian syndrome and subacute combined degeneration of the cord. Three new photographs appear illustrating rheumatoid involvement of the radio-ulnar joint.

Acknowledgments

MISS CASH would like to express her thanks to all the contributors for their interest and hard work in revising the various sections of this book. She would also like to thank Miss D. Caney, Principal, School of Physiotherapy, Queen Elizabeth Hospital, Birmingham, for her advice and for permission to use the School Library; Mrs. H. A. Atkinson, Principal, School of Physiotherapy, The Coventry and Warwickshire Hospital, and Miss C. M. Johnson, School of Physiotherapy, Royal Orthopaedic Hospital, Birmingham, for their help in Part IV; Miss P. Jean Cunningham, Editor of Nursing and Medical Books, Faber & Faber Ltd., for her time, help and advice in the preparation of this book.

The following would also like to express their thanks:

Miss D. Allen who wrote the chapter on Cerebral Palsy would like to thank the paediatricians and orthopaedic surgeons of St. Thomas's Hospital, the Director of the Physical Medicine Department and the Principal of the Physiotherapy School, the staff and patients of the Cerebral Palsy Unit, the Photographic Department of St. Thomas's Hospital, Dr. and Mrs. Bobath, the Western Cerebral Palsy Centre, London, and Miss Margaret Knott, Vallejo, California.

Miss E. A. Beazley who wrote the chapters on Diseases of the Respiratory System would like to thank Dr. D. Ahmad, L.M., L.R.C.P.I., L.R.C.S.I.

Miss B. Kennedy who wrote Physiotherapy in Paediatrics would like to thank Dr. Clive Shields, B.M., B.CH., Mr. Dudley Churchill-Davidson, M.A., M.B. B.CH., F.R.C.S., and Mrs. H. Angus, M.C.S.P. for their help and Miss J. Underhill, photographer to St. George's Hospital, for the photographs.

Miss F. McIlwraith who wrote Traumatic Lesions of the Spinal Cord would like to thank Sir Ludwig Guttmann, C.B.E., M.D., F.R.C.P., Consultant and Director of Research, National Spinal Injuries Centre, Stoke Mandeville Hospital, Miss D. T. Bell, M.C.S.P., formerly Superintendent Physiotherapist of Stoke Mandeville Hospital and Miss B. M. Graveling, M.C.S.P., Superintendent Physiotherapist at the Norfolk and Norwich Hospital, for their help.

Mrs. R. Smith who wrote three chapters in the section on Disorders of the Nervous System would like to thank Miss Sato, M.C.S.P., Superintendent Physiotherapist, National Hospital for Nervous Diseases, Queen

Square, and Mr. Reynolds, M.C.S.P., Superintendent Physiotherapist, Queen Mary's Hospital for Children, Carshalton.

Miss T. Wareham who wrote Hemiplegia would like to thank the Chest and Heart Association for permission to use drawings and material from their pamphlet *Return to Independence*.

Mrs. J. Wilhelm would like to thank Dr. Boyle, Miss Duffield and Miss Bartholomew for help with her chapters on Rheumatic Diseases, and Mr. D. R. Sweetman, M.A., B.A., M.B., B.CH., F.R.C.S., for three photographs showing attrition rupture of the extensor tendons due to rheumatoid involvement.

Contents

List of Contributors

Doreen Allen, S.R.N., M.C.S.P., DIP.T.P.
Member of Council and Physiotherapist to the Riding Centre for the Disabled, Chigwell

E. A. Beazley, M.C.S.P., DIP.T.P.
formerly Deputy Superintendent Physiotherapist, Lord Mayor Treloar Hospital, Alton, now at the School of Physiotherapy, the Middlesex Hospital, London W.1

Barbara Kennedy, M.C.S.P.
Superintendent Physiotherapist, Paediatric Department, St. George's Hospital, Tooting Grove

F. McIlwraith, M.C.S.P.
Assistant Superintendent Physiotherapist, St. Luke's Hospital, Guildford

Margaret Potter, M.C.S.P.
Superintendent Physiotherapist, Nuffield Orthopaedic Centre, Headington, Oxford

Rosemary Smith, M.C.S.P.
Former Physiotherapist with Dr. Kabat, Miriam Hospital, Providence, Rhode Island, U.S.A.

Margaret Stewart, F.C.S.P., DIP.T.P.
Principal of the School of Physiotherapy, King's College Hospital, Denmark Hill, London S.E.5

Truda Wareham, M.C.S.P., DIP.T.P.
formerly Superintendent Physiotherapist, St. Bartholomew's Hospital

Jean Wilhelm, M.C.S.P.
Senior Physiotherapist, Middlesex Hospital

List of Plates

List of Figures

PART I

Pathological Changes

CHAPTER 1

Inflammation and Healing

INFLAMMATION IS THE RESPONSE of the body to injury and has been defined as 'the reaction of vascular and supporting elements of the tissue which results in the formation of a protein-rich exudate, and is caused by injury, provided the injury has not been so severe as to destroy the area'. (Walter and Israel.)

CAUSES

Any factor which damages the cells sets up the process of inflammation. Such factors may be mechanical injury in accidents—dislocations, contusions, lacerations; chemical agents such as corrosive acids and alkalis; viruses and bacteria; physical agents including excessive heat or cold; injury due to ischaemia or hormone deficiency.

CHANGES

These occur in the calibre of arterioles, venules and capillaries; in the walls of the vessels and the rate of blood flow within them. They result in fluid and cellular exudation. There are also changes in the other components of the damaged tissues.

Vascular response

The immediate response to injury is vasoconstriction due to direct mechanical stimulation of the capillaries. This is rapidly followed by dilatation of arterioles, venules and capillaries, and opening up of small vessels which were not carrying blood at the moment of injury. Dilatation of the capillaries is the result of chemical substances. In the early stages histamine produces the dilatation, later many substances have been thought to be responsible, but there is still uncertainty as to which of these is really important. There are probably a variety of proteolytic enzymes and polypeptides concerned. Dilatation of the arterioles results from stimulation of the axon reflex.

The increase in the lumen of the vessels means an increase in the rate of blood flow, but this is quickly followed by slowing and stasis because of (i) the increased viscosity of the blood resulting from the loss of fluid into the intercellular spaces, (ii) the increase in peripheral resistance. When the vessels are normal the blood cells occupy the centre of the stream and there is a clear zone of plasma adjacent to the walls of the vessels. This decreases the viscosity of the blood flowing in the vessels and therefore lessens resistance. When the tissues are damaged the endothelial cells swell and become coated with a gelatinous substance of uncertain origin and the red cells run into rouleaux, displacing the lighter white cells into the clear zone. These cells then adhere to the sticky endothelium. Platelets also tend to adhere and little masses of white cells and platelets form and may even occlude the lumen. Thus thrombosis of small vessels is quite possible. The adherence of the white cells to the vessel walls is known as *margination*.

Exudation. Both fluid and cells pass into the tissues. The passage of fluid is due to the upset of balance between the hydrostatic and osmotic pressures of the blood. Normally fluid is driven out from the capillaries by the hydrostatic pressure and is attracted back by the osmotic pressure exerted by the plasma proteins. When damage occurs the capillaries become more permeable and more fluid containing the plasma proteins, which normally do not pass through the endothelial cells, passes into the tissues. The intercellular fluid has, therefore, a higher osmotic pressure and less fluid is attracted back. In addition metabolic processes in the tissue are speeded up and the consequent breakdown of large protein molecules into smaller ones further increases the osmotic pressure of the intercellular fluid. Alteration also occurs in the ground substance of the tissues and they become more fluid. This allows the exudate to diffuse more widely so that tension does not rise so rapidly in the tissues. An immediate rise in tension would tend to prevent fluid exudation.

The increase in *fluid exudation* with a high specific gravity and high protein content is important because it dilutes toxic agents; brings anti-bacterial substances and antibodies and also antibiotics and drugs, if these have been administered and have entered the blood stream. It also brings with it phagocytic cells. Since the fluid has a high protein content it tends to clot. A fibrin network is formed which prevents the spread of harmful agents and provides a scaffolding for the movement of phagocytic cells and for the growth of new tissues if this is necessary.

Cellular exudation is also important. Phagocytic cells pass out of the capillaries by pushing their way between the cells and then bursting through the basement membrane. This is known as the *process of emigration*. The first cells to pass out are the *neutrophils*. These are followed by the larger slower moving *monocytes*, usually known when they reach the tissue spaces as *macrophages*. The cells move towards the damaged area. It is not certain whether this is simply a random movement or whether they are attracted by products released by the injured tissues or bacteria. The neutrophils ingest damaged cells and bacteria, and then start the process of digestion. They have only a short life of two to three days, and any undigested particles which are liberated into the intercellular fluid on the death of these cells, together with tissue debris, are removed by the macrophages. In many cases of inflammation some red cells leave the capillaries. They follow the white cells simply by being ejected through the gaps made by these cells under the influence of the hydrostatic pressure of the blood. This process is known as *diapedesis*, a term originally applied to the passage of the white cells, but now more commonly used for the red cell ejection.

Changes in other components of the damaged tissues. An early and important change is in the groundwork of the tissues. This changes from a gel to a fluid so preventing early rise in tissue tension and allowing diffusion of the excess fluid.

CHANGES WHICH FOLLOW

If the injury has not caused much destruction the first change is the removal of fibrin, dead and damaged white cells, red cells, bacteria and any foreign material. This is done by the macrophages.

Excess fluid is removed in two ways. Some flows back into the capillaries because, with the removal of the irritant, the vessels return to normal and the balance between hydrostatic and osmotic pressures is restored. Much of the fluid is carried by the lymphatics to the regional lymph nodes, where cellular debris is dealt with by the cells lining the sinuses. Undamaged polymorphs pass back into the blood and lymph streams and macrophages wander back into the surrounding connective tissues. When these changes are complete, inflammation is resolved, and the damaged area returns to its original state. This is known as *resolution*.

Occasionally the process of removal of exudate is slow in which case granulation tissue grows into the fibrin clot and the ultimate result is fibrosis of the area. This often occurs in inflammation of serous membranes and results in the formation of adhesions which tend to develop in pleurisy and pericarditis. This is probably because the extensive fibrinous exudate is more than the macrophages can deal with and some of it becomes converted into fibrous tissue.

Should considerable tissue destruction result from the harmful agent, resolution is not possible and *suppuration* occurs. If the causative agents are micro-organisms, there is liberation of toxins which cause necrosis of tissue cells. In addition, whatever the cause, the stasis in the small blood vessels may interfere with the circulation sufficiently to bring about death of cells at the centre of the lesion. The immediate response to this is profuse infiltration of the area by polymorphs, which are attacked by the micro-organisms and many destroyed. Protein-splitting enzymes are released from the dead polymorphs and tissue cells. The enzymes digest the dead tissue and the fibrin produced by clotting of the exudate, and the necrotic tissue is softened and liquefied. The resulting fluid is pus, and the cavity in which it is contained is known as the *abscess*. Pus is liquid containing dead and dying white cells, inflammatory exudate and fibrin, dead and living micro-organisms and the products of tissue break-down, nucleic acids and lipids. The pus tends to track in the line of least resistance until it reaches and breaks through a free surface. When the pus is able to discharge either this way, or preferably by surgical interference, the cavity will heal by granulation tissue unless a chronic infection develops. In this case more pus is formed, the walls of the cavity become thickened by fibrous tissue and pus persistently discharges so that a *sinus* develops.

Occasionally the abscess fails to discharge and pus becomes walled off with thick fibrous tissue. Gradually fluid is absorbed and the pus thickens into a porridge-like consistency. Occasionally it becomes calcified.

SIGNS AND SYMPTOMS

Inflammation is characterised by redness, heat, pain, swelling and loss of function. Should there be suppuration there follows rise of temperature, respiration and pulse rate, together with other signs of fever.

Redness is due to the vascular dilatation and consequent hyperaemia. Dilatation of the capillaries produces a dull red area, dilatation of arterioles a brighter red flare. This can be seen if the skin is firmly stroked with a hard object. The immediate response is a white line caused by temporary vasoconstriction. This is followed by a dull red line which is rapidly surrounded by a bright red flare. The dull red area then swells and a *wheal* may appear due to the exudate causing the red line to become paler. This is the triple response of the skin to injury described by Lewis.

Heat. Dilatation of arterioles increases the blood supply to the part. If the temperature of the affected area is lower than that of the blood because the area is in contact with the external environment, the increased blood flow will raise its temperature. Heat is not felt in deeper tissues for this reason and because the organs do not have heat-sensitive nerve endings.

Pain. This is at least partly due to tension created in the tissues by the exudate. It will therefore be greatest if there is little room for swelling, resulting in greater pressure on pain-sensitive nerve endings. It may be that pain is also the result of concentration of hydrogen ions in an inflamed area or due to chemical substances liberated by damaged tissues.

Swelling. Inflammatory exudate accumulating in the affected area produces swelling, the amount depending on the severity of the inflammatory changes, the tension of the particular tissues and the extent to which the fluid can diffuse away. It may also be due to increased activity of special secreting cells involved in the injury. Thus if a synovial membrane is inflamed there will be inflammatory exudate causing swelling of the membrane and increased synovial fluid producing an effusion into the joint cavity.

Loss of function. Inflammation will upset the functions of the tissues. For example if a joint is inflamed it is painful and there will be reflex inhibition of the muscles acting on the joint. Swelling would also make movement difficult.

HEALING

The fundamental process of healing is the formation of granulation tissue. It occurs in the healing of wounds, the repair of ruptured tendons, the healing of fractured bones and, in fact, in the repair of all tissues. The final result is either regeneration or repair. *Regeneration* is the replacement of lost tissue by similar tissue and occurs when the cells of the damaged tissue are capable of division. *Repair* is replacement by scar tissue where the cells are unable to regenerate and granulation tissue is converted into scar tissue.

STAGES OF HEALING

Inflammation. However slight the injury some cells will be destroyed and there is often also haemorrhage. This sets up inflammation with fluid and cellular exudation. Blood and fluid clot and fibrin is formed.

Removal of debris. Phagocytic cells infiltrate the area, protein-splitting enzymes are liberated and dead cells and necrotic tissue are softened and liquefied.

Granulation tissue. The connective tissue elements begin to proliferate. The endothelial cells of the surrounding capillaries multiply and form buds which rapidly develop a lumen, forming loops through which the blood flows. Loops anastomose with one another and the new capillaries gradually extend into the area being cleared by the phagocytes. At first the new vessels are all capillaries but gradually some acquire a muscular coat to form arterioles and others enlarge to form venules. New lymphatics develop in the same way. At the same time fibroblasts grow with the capillaries into the area and gradually collagenous fibres form around them. It is not certain how these form but they only do so in the presence of fibroblasts. These cells are also thought to be responsible for the production of the ground substance of the new tissue.

While all this is going on, building materials collect in the area in the fluid exudate, and nerve fibres gradually grow into the granulation tissue.

Conversion into similar tissue or into scar tissue. If the cells of the damaged tissue can divide, new cells infiltrate the granulation tissue but if they cannot, the tissue becomes increasingly fibrous. The collagen fibres thicken and new layers are laid down at right angles to each other so that eventually a tough bundle or membrane of collagen fibre is formed. Tension on these fibres seems to determine the direction in which they lie. Meanwhile some of the new blood vessels begin to atrophy while others show such proliferation of the endothelium that their lumen is obliterated. As devascularisation and thickening increase, pale avascular scar tissue is formed. This has a great tendency to contract, thereby deforming the surrounding tissues.

RATE OF HEALING

This is influenced by both local and general factors.

Local factors. One of the most important of these is the blood supply. Poor circulation delays healing. The richness of the blood supply varies in different regions of the body. In addition circulation is impaired by prolonged pressure, as in bed sores. It is also decreased by oedema and reduced in chronic inflammation, since this is often accompanied by thickening of the intima and obliteration of the lumen of the blood vessels. Infection will always delay healing since the toxins produced by microorganisms destroy tissue. Persistent irritation will cause healing to be slowed, thus the presence of foreign bodies will have this effect. Continual breakdown of granulation tissue due to rough handling or repeated dressing of a wound will have a similar result.

Rate of healing is increased by physical measures which stimulate the circulation. Thus heat, ultraviolet light and moderate exercise will all help the healing process.

General factors. Young people heal quickly though age does not slow healing unless atheroma is present. Protein starvation, Vitamin C deficiency and excessive corticosteroids all delay healing, since they interfere with the formation of collagen. Healing is slowed by cold.

HEALING OF SKIN WOUNDS

Clean wounds without tissue loss. (First intention healing.) The small gap in the tissues is filled with blood which rapidly clots. An inflammatory reaction occurs at the edges of the wound and fluid exudate is added to the clot. The fibrin binds the edges together. Phagocytes immediately invade the clotted exudate and start to remove the fibrin and debris. Within twenty-four hours capillary buds and fibroblasts grow out from the surrounding tissue and meet across the exudate. Gradually collagen fibres are laid down and devascularised granulation tissue joins the sides of the wound. While all this is going on epithelial cells have been proliferating. These migrate into the wound and their presence appears to stimulate the growth of granulation tissue. As the tissue grows the cells are pushed upwards to cover the surface.

With this type of wound little granulation tissue is needed to fill the gap and practically no scar tissue results.

Wounds with tissue loss. (Healing by second intention.) There is no real difference in the healing process except that there is an actual gap which has to be filled, more granulation tissue is therefore formed and more scar tissue results. The gap is filled by clotted exudate and blood. Phagocytic cells invade the clot. Capillaries and fibroblasts grow in from the sides and floor of the wound, filling it with granulation tissue. Epithelial cells at the edges of the wound multiply and migrate down the sides into the wound between the connective tissue and the clot, forcing the latter up. As the granulation tissue grows up from the floor and sides, the 'tongues' of epithelial cells growing down on the edges of the gap are forced up until they cover the surface. Should there be much loss of epithelium, cells are obtained from the bases of the hair follicles and sweat glands. The granulation tissue gradually becomes avascular and eventually scar tissue is formed.

HEALING OF OTHER SOFT TISSUES

Healing of damaged tendons takes place in an identical way to that of burns except that tendon cells are found in the granulation tissue and very slowly regeneration will occur. If the ends of the tendon are not joined, however, union will be by fibrous tissue and the danger is then that repeated stretching due to movement will elongate the fibrous tissue, lengthening the tendon and reducing power.

In a minor injury of a muscle with rupture of individual fibres, regeneration can occur but in more severe injuries scar tissue forms. Cardiac muscle fibres have no ability to divide, consequently damage to the heart muscle is healed by fibrous tissue—an infarct is converted into fibrous tissue. Nerve tissue within the brain and spinal cord has no power of regeneration since nerve cells cannot reproduce and axons can only grow if there is a neurilemma, and nerve fibres in the central nervous system do not have a neurilemmal sheath. Peripheral nerves on the other hand can regenerate if the cells of origin of the axons are still intact.

HEALING OF BONE

Bone can reproduce itself because its special cells can multiply. The general process of healing is identical with other tissues but there is a source of bone-forming cells in the periosteum, bone and endosteum and in addition calcium salts are available. The stages of healing are therefore: haemorrhage and inflammation beneath the stripped-up periosteum, in the medullary cavity and between the bone ends; clotting of blood and exudate forming a soft mass between and around the bone ends; infiltration by neutrophils, and macrophages and osteoclasts to remove debris including dead fragments of bone; formation of granulation tissue by growth into the clot of capillaries, fibroblasts and osteoblasts; the formation of trabeculae of bone by the osteoblasts in the granulation tissue, hardening the mass which is then known as *Callus*. During these stages the pH of the blood has decreased—the acid tide—and calcium salts are absorbed from the blood. By about the tenth day the pH has risen above normal level—the alkaline tide—and calcium salts are now deposited in the callus, hardening it still further. Gradually the callus under the influence of osteoblasts and osteoclasts becomes converted into bone and remodelling occurs until the healing process has brought the bone back to its normal structure.

CHRONIC INFLAMMATION

This type of inflammation is characterised by the formation of fibrous tissue causing thickening, loss of elasticity and pliability of the tissues and disturbance of function.

Chronic inflammation is either due to the persistence of the agent which initiated acute inflammation or to an agent which has caused so mild a reaction that it has not been recognised. In the former case a foreign body may not have been removed by the acute reaction; the body's defensive mechanism to a particular micro-organism such as the tubercle bacillus may be low; the factors which delay healing may be present. In the latter case certain micro-organisms produce only a fleeting acute reaction but tend to remain in the tissues causing chronic irritation. The tubercle bacillus is an illustration of this type of bacterium. Pneumoconiosis (the disease produced by inhalation of dust) is another illustration. Asbestos workers inhale particles of asbestos. These particles are too large to be removed by the macrophages so they remain in the alveoli, stimulate a mild reaction which is followed by extensive fibrosis of the lung.

Two types of chronic inflammation therefore are found: that which follows acute inflammation and that in which there has been no appreciable preceding acute reaction. There is little difference between the changes which occur in the two types so they will be considered together.

CHANGES

Changes are a mixture of the vascular and exudative changes of inflammation, the attempt to clear the debris and micro-organisms, and the processes of healing. There is the state in which inflammation and healing are going on at the same time.

In many cases of chronic inflammation there is extensive exudation of protein-rich fluid leading to the production of considerable quantities of fibrin. This is particularly seen in chronic, suppurative inflammation and inflammation of serous sacs. Many cells are in the area including large quantities of macrophages which may have fused to form giant cells. These cells are softening and removing the dead cells and debris. Lymphocytes and plasma cells are found in great numbers. The function of the latter cells is uncertain but they are a feature of the granulation tissue in chronic inflammation. Endothelial cells are also present forming new capillaries. These are especially noticeable in the lining of chronic abscess cavities and they break down readily leading to haemorrhage.

Fibroblasts are present in large numbers and lay down the collagen which produces a large quantity of fibrous tissue. If the cells of the chronically inflamed tissue can divide then regeneration occurs. Quite often there is excessive production of new cells, this is particularly noticeable in epithelial tissues.

SIGNS AND SYMPTOMS

These depend on the area involved. Fibrous tissue replacing specialised tissue cannot carry out the functions of the tissue in which it is formed. It may, for example, form adhesions binding the lung to the chest wall and interfering with expansion; it may 'stick' ligaments to the bones over which they pass, limiting movement; it may bind tendons in their sheaths and interfere with the work of muscles. It can reduce the elasticity of tubes as in chronic bronchitis and, replacing glands, reduce secretions.

Chronic suppurative inflammation may give rise to haemorrhage as in stomach ulcers and it always gives rise to general symptoms of loss of appetite, loss of weight, anaemia, headache and tiredness.

CHAPTER 2

Thrombosis. Embolism. Oedema

THROMBOSIS

A THROMBUS IS A SOLID BODY formed in the cardiovascular system from the constituents of blood. Blood platelets adhere to the lining of the vessel, thromboplastin is liberated and fibrin is formed and deposited on the little mass of platelets. More platelets then adhere and some white and red cells are trapped in the fibrinous network. The mass gradually or quickly (depending on the speed of blood flow, slowly if flow is quick and thromboplastin is swept away) builds up until it occludes the lumen of the vessel. If a vein is involved stasis then occurs proximal to the thrombus and the blood therefore clots to the point at which the next tributary vein joins the affected vein. Propagation of the clot may then occur because the proximal end of the clot may present a rough surface and platelets from the incoming blood start to adhere, clotting then develops proximally to the entry of the next tributary. Eventually a clot one or two feet long may form.

Later changes in the thrombus. Capillary buds and fibroblasts grow into the solid mass from the deeper layers of the vessel wall while phagocytic cells remove the cellular content. Thus the thrombus becomes firmly adherent to the vessel. At this point it is unlikely to be displaced though the proximal clot is not thus organised and can break off. If the vessel wall is inflamed adherence will develop more rapidly since inflammation is characterised by the growth of granulation tissue.

A second change which occurs is canalisation of the thrombus. Endothelial cells multiply and grow into the thrombus between the strands of fibrin, while the macrophages are removing the red and white cells. In this way channels are formed in the thrombus and blood can flow through it.

CAUSES

The deposit of platelets is the main feature in thrombosis and this may occur in three circumstances: changes in the endothelial lining of the vessel; slowing of the blood flow; eddy currents which deflect the platelets to the walls of the vessels.

Changes in the endothelium so that it no longer presents a smooth shiny state may result from vascular disease; from direct injury in accidents and surgery; from anoxia; from pressure or from chemical irritants. Kinking of the vessel due to neighbouring scar contracture will affect the endothelium and it will also cause eddy currents.

Slowing of blood flow will occur in any medical illness, accident or surgery which demands the patient being confined to bed for even a short time, and from congestive heart failure. At normal speed the cellular content of the blood travels at the centre of the stream leaving a clear plasmatic zone near the walls of the vessel. With slowing of flow the platelets and white cells fall out into the clear zone and are therefore more likely to adhere to the endothelium.

Other factors may also increase the danger of thrombus formation. If the number of platelets rises they appear to become more sticky and therefore more likely to adhere. The platelet number is known to increase following trauma and haemorrhage. There is therefore a rise following surgery and childbirth.

Age, obesity, blood changes such as raised erythrocyte sedimentation rate, reduced fibrinogen content, may all play a part. Thrombosis is more common in elderly patients and in obese people.

SITE

Thrombosis can occur in any part of the vascular system. In the *arteries* it may develop due to various factors: injury such as could be produced by sharp spicules of bone in a fracture; inflammation as in thrombo-angiitis obliterans; degenerative disease as in arterio-sclerosis; dilatation of arterial walls giving rise to an aneurysm. These agents may produce spasm and slowing of blood flow; inflammatory changes in the endothelium leading to deposit of platelets; ulceration of the intima, or stasis in an aneurysm.

Thrombosis in the *heart* is the result of stasis such as may occur in mitral stenosis when a thrombus may form in the left auricle. Thrombi tend to develop on the heart valves in acute rheumatism which causes inflammation of the endocardium. The walls of the ventricles may be involved when there has been a myocardial infarction following coronary thrombosis.

The commonest site of thrombosis is in the *veins*. It is either due to inflammation of the vein due to injury, bacteria or the introduction of chemicals when it is known as a Thrombophlebitis, or it may be due to causes previously discussed, when it is termed Phlebothrombosis.

The latter type tends to complicate surgery and parturition because several causative agents are then present, including a rise in the number of platelets and amount of thromboplastin (the latter released from damaged tissue); slowing of blood flow due to inactivity and, in the case of abdominal and thoracic surgery, reduced respiratory excursion; minor damage to endothelium such as may well occur from pressure on the calves when the patient is unconscious.

EFFECTS OF THROMBOSIS

The effects of thrombosis will depend upon the vessel affected, the degree to which the mass occludes the lumen, and the state of the collateral vessels. Some thrombi are dissolved, probably the result of a plasminogen activator in the endothelium, others shrink and become canalised. Some may become detached and form emboli and effects then depend upon where the embolus becomes impacted. If collateral circulation is not rapidly established in arterial thrombosis, death of tissue occurs, the dead tissue is gradually softened by autolysins and protein-splitting enzymes, and replaced by granulation tissue from the surrounding unaffected tissue. The granulation tissue changes into fibrous tissue. Such an area is known as an infarct and its seriousness depends upon the ability of the undamaged tissue to do the work of the destroyed tissue.

The effect of thrombosis in veins has been fully described elsewhere (see *Physiotherapy in some Surgical Conditions*).

EMBOLISM

An embolus is a foreign body circulating in the blood stream. When it enters a vessel too small to allow it to pass, it becomes impacted and completely blocks the vessel producing a state of anaemia. Though the embolus is nearly always part or the whole of a detached thrombus, it can be a globule of fat derived from ruptured fat cells or it can be air. In the former case it is a complication of fractures in which the fat, in a liquid form, is released from the ruptured fat cells of the bone marrow and passes into the veins of the cancellous spaces. In the latter case air may enter the blood stream and so reach the heart where it becomes churned up with the blood, forming a frothy mass which interferes with the passage of blood through the heart. Emboli derived from a thrombus most often enter the venous circulation and so reach the right side of the heart to become impacted in the pulmonary circulation. Emboli formed in the left side of the heart may block the coronary or cerebral vessels.

Effect of embolism. Both thrombi and emboli block the vessels but the former usually produce a gradual blocking with a state of chronic anaemia. The effect of the latter is sudden, no time having been allowed for the dilatation of collateral vessels supplying the same area. In this case the result depends upon the presence of collateral vessels and the speed with which they open up. If the embolus impacts in a small vessel with many anastomosing branches, no ill effect may occur. If it obstructs a large vessel, such as the axillary artery, the limb would rapidly become cold, pulseless, cyanotic and oedematous. But warmth and colour would gradually return since blood can reach the limb through the branches of the sub-clavian artery, and provided these are healthy they will rapidly dilate. There may be some residual effects, but the health of the limb will be maintained. Should the obstruction occur in one of the main cerebral or coronary arteries which are entirely responsible for the nutrition of one area of the brain or heart, that area of tissue must inevitably undergo necrosis and infarction occurs.

DISTURBANCE OF THE FORMATION AND DRAINAGE OF TISSUE FLUID

OEDEMA

Oedema is the accumulation of fluid in the cells and fibres of the tissues and in the spaces between them. Its absorption into the cells and fibres renders the part firmer and heavier. Its presence in the tissue spaces may give rise to 'pitting on pressure'. If the area is firmly pressed on by the fingers or thumb, a pit or hollow is left when the fingers are removed; gradually the pit will fill again giving evidence that the swelling is a fluid one and that the fluid is under slight pressure.

NORMAL FORMATION OF TISSUE FLUID

Tissue fluid is formed under the influence of three main factors: hydro-static pressure, osmotic pressure and the permeability of the capillary walls.

Hydrostatic pressure. The blood pressure in the capillaries is higher than the pressure of the tissue fluid, consequently blood plasma filters through the capillary wall into the tissues.

Osmotic pressure. The osmotic pressure of the blood is largely dependent upon the plasma proteins, particularly upon the serum albumin. The capillary wall is, under normal circumstances, not permeable to these

c

proteins, consequently the osmotic pressure of the capillary blood is greater than that of the tissue fluid. An attractive force is therefore exerted to withdraw the fluid from the tissue space.

Permeability of the capillary wall. The capillary endothelium is permeable to certain substances and not to others. Water, glucose and salts may all pass through, provided they are in greater concentration on one side of the membrane than the other. Plasma proteins cannot normally diffuse through the endothelial cells. This fact tends to keep the osmotic pressure of the blood high and that of the tissue fluid lower. This permeability can be altered. Any factor which brings about dilatation of the capillary will also increase the permeability of its cells, and it is then that plasma proteins may enter the tissue fluid.

Under normal circumstances a balance is kept between the fluid which is formed and that which is absorbed. Fluid passes into the tissues under the influence of the hydrostatic pressure and is attracted back under the influence of the osmotic pressure. The fluid which does not return to the blood filters through into the lymph capillaries under pressure from the tissue fluid. The quantity of fluid varies with rest and exercise. Activity of the muscles brings about vaso-dilatation and increased formation of metabolites. Vaso-dilatation results in increased formation of tissue fluid, while increased metabolites may raise the osmotic pressure of the tissue fluid, so that the attractive force of the capillary blood is lessened. The stiffness which follows strenuous exercise is the result of increased fluid in the tissue space.

FACTORS RESPONSIBLE FOR OEDEMA

Alteration in any or all of the three factors will result in excessive tissue fluid formation. As the lymph vessels also help to carry away tissue fluid, any obstruction in the lymphatic drainage will have the same effect. In addition, the flow of venous blood and lymph may be impaired since it is dependent on joint movement, muscle contractions and the suction action of the low intrathoracic pressure.

Increase in hydrostatic pressure. This will, if it is sufficiently prolonged, cause oedema. It is usually not the only cause, since a rise in hydrostatic pressure in the capillaries means a disturbance of the circulation with change in the endothelium and increased permeability. A rise in hydrostatic pressure may be the result of general or local factors. If the heart fails to maintain a normal circulation there will be congestion in the veins and hydrostatic pressure will rise in the capillaries. Increased filtration will therefore occur. An obstruction in a large vein will have exactly the same effect though it will be localised to the area which is drained by that vein.

Fall in osmotic pressure. This will lessen the attractive force exerted by the blood and fluid will tend to accumulate in the tissues. A fall in the osmotic pressure may be the result of one type of kidney disease which results in a greater quantity of plasma proteins being lost through the kidney. It may arise because the permeability of the capillary wall is increased and plasma proteins pass into the intercellular fluid.

The plasma proteins may also be deficient, as a result of starvation, and a nutritional oedema may develop.

Increased capillary permeability. Trauma or nutritional disturbances may alter the permeability of the endothelium. A capillary reacts to irritation not only by dilating but also by changes in the endothelial lining. A great quantity of fluid may enter the tissues as a result of this factor both in severe lacerations and in burns. Any factor which disturbs the nutrition of the cells will also increase their permeability. If the blood is circulating unduly slowly, it loses oxygen and gains more than the normal carbon dioxide. This disturbs the physical state of the endothelium and tissue fluid increases. Oedema will therefore occur, not only following trauma but also in all cases of venous congestion.

Lymphatic obstruction. Tissue fluid may be formed normally but its drainage may be impaired, either because it is not adequately absorbed into the venous end of the capillary because hydrostatic pressure is too high or osmotic pressure too low, or because the lymph channels are blocked. Lymph vessels may be blocked by the action of parasites, as a result of inflammation, by pressure of tumours or scar tissue, or as a result of surgical stripping. Lymphatic glands into which the lymph vessels drain may themselves be involved, either as a result of disease processes such as carcinoma or because their removal is a surgical necessity.

Slowed flow of blood and lymph. Weak or paralysed muscles, stiff joints and poor action of the diaphragm will all reduce the venous and lymphatic return so that tissue drainage is impaired.

EFFECTS OF OEDEMA

The presence of extensive oedema is liable to set up an arterial spasm and so cause an anaemic condition of the area. Even if it fails to cause spasm it causes anaemia because, as the hydrostatic pressure of the tissue fluid rises, pressure is exerted on the capillaries and arterial inflow is retarded.

Persistent fluid in the tissue spaces interferes with the nutrition of the cells since fresh nutrient substances and gases are not available and waste products are not removed; metabolism is therefore seriously impaired.

Atrophy, loss of tone and elasticity, and defective resistance and healing properties must all inevitably result. The function of the area is therefore impaired.

In the course of time, the fluid will tend to organise into fibrous tissue and the area becomes indurated and hardened. The speed with which this occurs depends upon the characteristics of the oedema fluid. If it contains a high percentage of protein it will clot readily. This condition exists when the fluid is largely the result of increased capillary permeability and is less likely when the major factor in its formation is either raised hydrostatic pressure or low osmotic pressure. Should the fluid clot, it forms a mass foreign to the tissues and they will react by proliferation. Cells and blood vessels invade the clotted fluid and it gradually becomes converted into fibrous tissue. This may have serious results because the fibrous tissue tends to shrink. As it shrinks it may obliterate blood vessels, so causing anaemia and gross disturbance in local nutrition. It may, if it has occurred in the periarticular structures, cause limitation of movement in joints. Should the fluid have invaded muscles, pliability and extensibility will be impaired. Muscular contraction may be seriously hampered by the presence of scar tissue. Should oedema occur in serous membranes, adhesions may form resulting in interference with the movements of the underlying organs.

In addition to all these ill-effects, the presence of fluid distending the tissue spaces is a source of permanent discomfort and annoyance to the patient.

TYPES OF OEDEMA

Oedema occurs in many different conditions; often therefore a special name is used to indicate the type. Cardiac, renal and starvation oedema are examples of a generalised oedema. Local oedema is probably more common, and traumatic, obstructive, paralytic, and oedema due to poor muscle tone and laxity of fascia are illustrations of this type. In each, one or other of the factors previously discussed are responsible.

Cardiac oedema. While largely due to the rise in hydrostatic pressure in the capillaries, following failure of the heart to maintain a normal circulation, it may also be due to the low oxygen tension in the blood causing increased permeability of the capillary walls. The fluid formed has, therefore, a high protein content and will clot and organise. Until it clots it will pit on pressure.

The oedema of this type is found first in the periphery where circulation is the slowest, and it tends to gather in the most dependent areas. If the patient is up it will be seen therefore in the feet and around the ankles, gradually spreading up the legs. If the patient is in bed it will be seen also in the abdomen and sacral region. The quantity of fluid is always greatest at night, when the heart is tired, and least in the morning.

Renal oedema. This is the result of either a drop in osmotic pressure or a decrease in capillary permeability according to the disease affecting the kidney. In the first case the fluid will have a low specific gravity since its protein content is small; in the second case the protein content and, therefore, the specific gravity will be high. Since this oedema does not depend on venous congestion and slowing of the circulation it will not collect in the periphery nor will it be worse at night. It is often noticeable in the face, particularly in the lax tissue around the eyes, and is worse in the morning; it tends to be dispersed during the day by muscular action.

Starvation oedema. This is probably partly the result of a drop in the osmotic pressure of the blood as a result of a deficiency of proteins, partly due to nutritional disturbances of the endothelium resulting in increasing permeability, and partly to decreased heart action and slowing of the circulation.

Traumatic oedema. One of the most serious results of extensive burns is the great loss of fluid into the tissues. In a lesser degree this is also seen in injuries such as extensive lacerations, fractures and dislocations. Various factors enter into this type of oedema. Local hydrostatic pressure rises because the irritation of the sensory nerve endings and the release of a histamine-like substance brings about extensive vaso-dilatation and hyperaemia. The injury also causes great increase in the permeability of the dilated capillaries. Lymphatic vessels and veins are also injured and possibly thrombosed with interference with the drainage of tissue fluid. Drainage is also impaired because damage usually implies diminished function, and the pumping effect on these soft-walled vessels of the muscular contractions and joint movements is either reduced or lost.

The fluid formed has a very high protein content and clots and organises readily. For this reason the final effects on the area may be serious if care is not taken.

Obstructive oedema. This develops if either venous or lymphatic obstruction occurs. This may be the result of deep venous thrombosis, lymphangitis, pressure of scars or tumours or removal of lymph glands and vessels. In a condition such as phlegmasia alba dolens (white leg), femoral thrombosis and chronic inflammation of the lymph vessels are probably both responsible. The oedema following radical mastectomy is an illustration of obstructive oedema which may be due to removal of lymph glands or to pressure by axillary scar tissue. The presence of fluid is mainly due to a rise in hydrostatic pressure and the fluid will have a low protein content and will clot only slowly. Nevertheless in the course of time it will organise.

Paralytic oedema. Oedema tends to result from muscular paralysis provided the vaso-dilators are not paralysed. In the latter case the vaso-constrictors are overactive and a cold limb results rather than oedema. When oedema occurs it is the result of either paralysis of the vaso-con-strictors causing widespread vaso-dilatation, congestion and increased filtration, or it may be the result of decreased function and loss of the pumping effect normally exerted on the veins and lymphatics. If the circulation is slowed as a result of either or both of these factors, the oxygen tension of the blood will fall and the capillaries will therefore become more permeable. The fluid is likely to have a high protein content and will readily organise.

Oedema due to poor muscle tone and laxity of fascia. In the erect position, venous blood from the legs and abdomen has to return to the heart against the force of gravity. It would therefore have a tendency to stagnate in these regions if it were not for certain factors. In the first place, the deep fascia of the lower extremity is particularly strong and extensive and acts as a kind of elastic stocking to support the veins. Many of the muscles either insert directly into this fascia or send expansions to reinforce it. The fascia is affected either by prolonged recumbency or by immobilisation of the limb in a rigid support since the muscles inserting into it will become weaker and hypotonic and the fascia will become less tense.

In the second place the tone of the muscles of the legs and abdominal wall plays a very important part in the prevention of 'pooling' of blood, thus any factor which causes decrease in tone may lead to venous conges-tion. Thirdly, the vaso-motor mechanism causes an increase in the tone of the veins when the posture is changed from lying to standing, but if this mechanism has not been fully in use for a period of time, then, when it is required, it does not act as effectively as it should. Oedema, therefore, tends to occur when a patient first gets up after a long period in bed, particularly if the illness has been one, such as rheumatoid arthritis, in which the muscles have been directly affected and their strength and tone reduced. It will also develop when a plaster splint has been removed after a prolonged period of immobilisation. In each case the inadequately constricted or supported vessels tend to dilate, venous congestion develops and excess tissue fluid is formed, partly under the influence of a raised hydrostatic pressure and partly as a result of increased capillary permeability. The fluid will have a relatively high protein content and will clot readily.

Idiopathic oedema. There are a few people in whom oedema tends to develop without known cause. This is an hereditary oedema which has certain peculiar features. It affects women mainly and may involve one or both legs. No treatment appears to be effective. It causes no outstanding symptoms but it brings about an unsightly thickening of the legs.

CHAPTER 3

Atrophy and Hypertrophy.
Hypoplasia and Hyperplasia.
Neoplasia

ALTERATION IN THE SIZE of individual cells and fibres or of an organ as a whole is not uncommonly seen. Such alteration in size is invariably accompanied byalt erations in function and in many cases, though not in all, is the result of disturbance of nutrition. For any cell or fibre to maintain its normal size once it reaches full development, it must carry out its normal function, its metabolism must continue undisturbed and its nervous connections must remain intact. It follows that disturbance of any one of these factors may cause increase or decrease in size. In addition such factors as the influence of toxins, the effect of the secretion of ductless glands and interference with the blood supply must all be considered.

ATROPHY

This is diminution in size of tissues. If the term is applied to muscles or organs it refers to the specialised elements and not the supporting framework, although in certain cases the connective tissue may increase at the same rate or even faster than the atrophy of the histological cells. This increase of interstitial structures may be explained by the fact that the atrophied cells and fibres are probably receiving and using less nutrient products and oxygen and more are therefore available for the less specialised tissue.

Probably one of the commonest causes of atrophy is diminished function. It is often seen in limbs which have been immobilised for a period of time. This atrophy is due to impaired katabolism since decreased katabolic processes mean decreased anabolism and therefore decrease in size. Disuse atrophy, as this type is usually called, is seen not only in muscles but also in other tissues which have lost their function, such as the ovaries after the menopause.

Injuries and disease of joint are almost invariably accompanied by rapid and severe atrophy of the muscles acting on the affected joint. Such atrophy is usually much more profound than could possibly be accounted for by disuse. The probable explanation is that either sympathetic fibres are disturbed and nutrition consequently impaired, or that reflex atrophy is the result of irritation of sensory nerve endings and so messages pass to the spinal cord and thus to the lateral and anterior horns of grey matter resulting in inhibition of activity of the cells.

Atrophy is also seen in circulatory disturbances. A slow progressive diminution in the lumen of the main vessels of a limb means gradual cutting down of the nutrition to all the tissues of that part and all specialised cells and fibres consequently shrink in size. Involvement of skin, muscles, joint structures and bone is seen in advanced arterio-sclerosis and Buerger's disease.

Continuous pressure is responsible for atrophy, partly because it reduces the blood supply to the part and partly because it impairs function and so katabolism. The presence of a tumour is liable to lead to atrophy of the tissue on which it grows.

In disease of the lower motor neurone atrophy will be present in all structures supplied either by the damaged neurones or by any other nerve fibres running with them. Several explanations arise for this: in the first place since no nerve impulses can reach the motor-end plate there can be no muscle tone or power of contraction and the result is abolition of katabolic processes with consequent atrophy of muscle fibres. In the second place, the vaso-constrictor fibres running with the motor fibres are also liable to be involved and if this occurs paralytic vaso-dilatation results in circulatory stasis and impairment of nutrition to all the structures in the region. Such atrophy is serious because it is likely to continue over a long period and will therefore be followed by degeneration of the tissues and permanent impairment of function.

Most cases of atrophy are local but a generalised atrophy is seen in chronic starvation and in fevers. In the latter case the toxins stimulate protein metabolism and a rapid wasting takes place particularly in the muscles. It is probably also partly the result of impaired digestion and absorption.

Effects of Atrophy. The primary effect of atrophy is decreased function. In the case of muscular tissue power depends on number and size of fibres. While atrophy does not normally affect the number it does affect size and therefore muscle power is markedly reduced as a result of atrophy. In addition atrophy may mean loss of elasticity. This is particularly seen in the skin and may lead to limitation of function.

HYPERTROPHY

This is the increase in size of the specialised elements of a tissue. Increase in the quantity of the connective tissue such as is seen in some types of muscular dystrophy is not true hypertrophy. This change in size is always the result of increased functional demands except in those cases which are the result of overactivity of the ductless glands. An increased functional demand means increased katabolism, consequently increased building up and so increase in the size of cells and fibres. It may be physiological or pathological. Physiological hypertrophy is not associated with disease, it is well illustrated in the case of the pregnant uterus or in the muscles of the athlete. The muscular tissue in either case is called upon to do extra work and hypertrophy results. Pathological hypertrophy, as its name implies, is associated with disease. An example of such an occurrence is seen in hypertrophy of the heart. Stenosis of the mitral valve hinders the flow of blood from the left atrium and the result is an increase in the breadth and length of its fibres. A similar hypertrophy may be seen in the involuntary muscular coat of the stomach in stenosis of the pyloric sphincter. There is a limit to the amount to which any cell can hypertrophy and when this point is reached either hyperplasia results or the functional demand fails to be met.

Pathological hypertrophy is sometimes compensatory. One group of cells and fibres enlarges to take over the work which should be done by damaged or lost tissue. This may be seen in one lobe of a lung when the other lobes have been removed or in one kidney when the other becomes diseased and fails to function.

A different illustration of hypertrophy is seen in diseases of the pituitary gland in the adult when hyperfunction results in enlargement of the girth of the bone and in thickening of the connective tissues throughout the body.

Effects of Hypertrophy. With the exception of the last type of hypertrophy increased size means increased function. Hypertrophied muscles have always greater power than normal muscles, provided that it is the whole muscle which is hypertrophied and not only a few groups of its fibres.

HYPOPLASIA AND HYPERPLASIA

These should not be confused with atrophy and hypertrophy. The latter terms invariably refer to size, the former to number or quantity. Hypoplasia and hyperplasia most commonly occur before the tissues have reached maturity and are then developmental defects often of unknown origin. Hypoplasia means a decreased number of cells or fibres and may be the result of disturbance of the ductless glands controlling growth and development, such as is seen in the pituitary dwarf. Hyperplasia is an increase in the number of cells and fibres either the result of increased activity of ductless glands during the period of growth, or the result of increased functional demands which cannot be entirely met by hypertrophy. Hyperplasia of bone marrow very readily occurs on a demand for increased blood; division of liver cells results in hyperplasia of the liver if a section of that organ is surgically removed. It is possible that some hyperplasia of cardiac muscle tissue may take place but it is not a feature of voluntary muscle cells.

NEOPLASIA

This is too vast a subject to be dealt with fully in a textbook of this type, but since the physiotherapist has to treat patients suffering from tumours a brief description of some of the features of neoplasia has been included.

Like hyperplasia, neoplasia is an increase in the number of cells, but, unlike the former, the increase arises spontaneously or as a result of some abnormal stimulus, and once started it continues even though the stimulus has ceased. The new cells acquire new characteristics and as these cells divide the daughter cells take on these same new features. There are also usually differences in the size, structure and relationship of the cells to one another. They also lose the specialised functions of the cells from which they originated and appear to be mainly concerned with proliferation. Another peculiar feature is their power to multiply and form new masses at sites distal to their origin if they are carried away in the blood or lymph stream.

As the cells multiply they may form masses supported by connective tissue—the stroma—and blood vessels, producing a tumour, or they may spread rapidly into the surrounding tissues when no mass may form, or both may happen at the same time.

A peculiar feature of the tumour is its ability to divert to itself a large proportion of nutritive substances so that the rest of the tissues of the body suffer. Thus a tumour may grow to large proportions while the rest of the body wastes.

Tumours are often divided into benign and malignant though there may be no clear distinction between the two and a benign tumour may suddenly begin to become malignant.

A benign tumour grows slowly, it usually possesses a capsule and its cells do not invade the surrounding tissue. The arrangement of its cells closely resembles that of the surrounding tissues. While not normally affecting the general health of the patient it can have serious effects by blocking tubes or if it is growing in glandular tissue it can cause irritation and so increased secretions.

Benign epithelial tumours of surface epithelium are known as papilloma, of glandular tissue as adenoma. Benign connective tissue tumours are usually named according to the tissue on which they grow: fibroma; osteoma; chondroma; lipoma; haemangioma; lymphangioma; meningioma.

Malignant tumours usually grow much more quickly and consequently do not develop a capsule. The cells always invade the surrounding tissues following the tissue planes in the line of least resistance. Fascial sheaths tend to confine them and cartilage to resist them. They tend to invade both blood and lymph vessels where they spread along the walls and sometimes block the vessels. This tendency accounts for the metastases seen in malignancy. Little groups of cells may form emboli and are carried round in the circulation till they become impacted in the capillary network. Here they multiply and secondary deposits—metastases—are formed. If such emboli are travelling in the venous circulation or enter the venous stream via the thoracic lymphatic ducts the first capillary network will be in the lungs. Secondary growths in the lungs are therefore common. Emboli in the portal circulation will impact in the liver and cause metastasis here.

Malignant tumours produce many ill effects. They produce pressure and obstruction; they cause cachexia, loss of weight and general atrophy; they destroy tissue and may undergo secondary infection. Anaemia is a frequent feature and if surface epithelium is involved haemorrhage often occurs. Pain is a common feature with its effect on general health.

Malignant tumours of surface and glandular epithelium are known as carcinoma, while if connective tissue is involved the term sarcoma is applied, thus we hear of liposarcoma, fibrosarcoma, osteogenic sarcoma. Various terms have been used for malignant tumours of lymphoid tissue of which lymphatic leukaemia is one. All malignant tumours are cancers, this term being used because of their characteristic spread into surrounding tissues.

Though some malignant tumours can occur at any age, most tend to develop after the age of fifty and they seem to be slightly more common in men than in women, though some are peculiar to women and some to men.

The cause is not yet certain but certain points are becoming clearer. Some types of tumour are common in certain occupations, and certain agents appear to predispose a whole area of tissue to neoplasia. These agents are carcinogenic and may be chemical or physical. Chemical agents may be derived from coal tar and mineral oils. Workers using arsenic seem liable to develop cancer of the skin of the limbs and face, carcinoma of the lungs is more common in those whose occupation brings them in contact with hot tar fumes, nickel and asbestos, or in those who are heavy cigarette smokers. Physical agents which appear to predispose the tissues are radioactive elements, X-rays and strong ultraviolet radiations.

While chronic irritants probably do not themselves produce cancer they may promote neoplasia in a tissue already predisposed by a carcinogenic agent.

Hormones appear to have some influence on the growth of tumours. Some breast cancers appear to depend for their growth on oestrogen, progesterone and prolactin, and ovariectomy and bilateral adrenalectomy sometimes cause a temporary regression in such cancers. In recent years some lesions of epithelial surfaces have been recognised in which the cells show changes, but in which there is no true malignancy or invasion of surrounding tissues. If such lesions can be detected treatment can be instituted which may prevent development of neoplasia and loss of life. In this, for example, lies the importance of the taking of cervical smears, since such changed cells are shed, and trapped in the mucus of the cervix.

PHYSIOTHERAPY IN RELATION TO TUMOURS

All tumours are a contra-indication to physiotherapy but physical measures may be needed to help to relieve their effects or in the case of treatment of neoplasia by surgery. For example, a tumour may be causing obstruction of a bronchus giving rise to accumulation of secretions and collapse of an area of lung, and postural drainage and coughing may be essential. A bilateral adrenalectomy or a radical mastectomy will require routine pre- and post-operative physiotherapy. Exercises may be needed to strengthen muscles and improve posture following surgery to remove lymph nodes and soft tissues in the region of tumours, as in block neck resection in laryngopharyngectomy. The fact that the patient is or has been suffering from tumours does not affect physiotherapy in such cases.

CHAPTER 4

Principles of Treatment by Physiotherapy of Inflammation and Oedema

INFLAMMATION

A VERY GREAT PROPORTION of conditions treated by the physio-therapist are inflammatory in origin and a clear understanding of the principles of treatment is therefore essential.

ACUTE INFLAMMATION

The changes of acute inflammation occur for a very definite purpose and should not be impeded. The first great principle of treatment therefore is *rest*. If the affected area is allowed to rest, nature will perform her function. Movement and handling at this stage simply increase the irritation so that the various changes are exaggerated and cannot fulfil their purpose. Rest may be gained in various ways according to the site of the lesion. The patient may be confined to bed, the limb may be splinted or the upper extremity may be supported in a sling. The main requirement is support so that movement does not occur and muscle spasm is avoided.

On the other hand absolute rest must not be maintained for too long because, if the circulation is slowed by diminished movement, absorption of exudate is reduced and organisation into fibrous tissue is then likely. The second principle of treatment is therefore *maintenance of normal circulation in the part affected*. This principle should be considered as soon as the height of inflammation is reached. At this stage, the purpose of the inflammatory change having been gained, resolution can be aided by promoting rapid absorption and preventing organisation. Circulation, and, therefore, absorption, can be aided by many different measures, but the simplest and most effective is active exercise. No great range of movement is necessary to obtain these objects. If, for example, tearing of muscle fibres precludes early movement of the joint on which the muscle works, rhythmic contractions of the muscle in whatever support is being used, together with vigorous movements of other joints, will stimulate the circulation and prevent the sticky exudate from turning into fibrous tissue. In the case of an inflamed joint where movements might still be contra-indicated, tendons may be kept moving in their sheaths and the circulation be kept free in the joint structures by isometric work of all muscle groups acting on the joint.

In very severe trauma excessive changes tend to occur and blood from ruptured vessels may be added to the inflammatory exudate. In this excessive exudate and haemorrhage lies a danger—the blood and lymph vessels may be quite incapable of removing the extravasated fluid. If seen at once, steps may be taken to prevent this state of affairs, and *a third principle is the prevention of excessive exudate and bleeding*. Putting the part at rest immediately partly fulfils this principle; some measure to stop haemorrhage and constrict vessels may also help. Ice, pressure bandages or evaporating lotions are suitable means.

In acute inflammation particularly affecting joint structures, atrophy of muscle occurs very rapidly. *It is essential to keep the atrophy as slight as possible* because the first line of defence of the joint will be impaired if muscles are weak and atrophied. Because of its origin it is impossible to prevent all atrophy, yet muscles may be maintained in a reasonable condition by massage and active exercises. Both measures are used with care, and massage is omitted and exercises are rapidly increased as in-flammation subsides.

From the physiotherapist's point of view, four main principles therefore stand out in the treatment of any acute inflammatory condition. They are: rest, prevention of excessive exudate, promotion of rapid absorption and prevention of organisation of exudate, and maintenance of muscle bulk and tone. It is immaterial whether the inflammation is that of a joint, as in rheumatoid arthritis, or an inflammation of fibrous tissue as in acute fibrositis, or of an organ as in pneumonia, the same principles apply, difference existing only in their method of application.

CHRONIC INFLAMMATION

As in the acute case, the physiotherapist must consider the changes which have occurred. The capsule or synovial membrane or other tissues may be thickened by the formation of new fibrous tissue; there may be anaemia, as permanently dilated vessels become thickened and blood-flow stagnates; part of the tissue may be adherent. As a result of these changes, movement is probably limited and muscles in the region grossly atrophied. The main objects of treatment can be clearly gathered from these facts. It is necessary to soften the indurated area and separate out the adherent tissues, to stretch the contracting fibrous tissues and to stretch or break down fibrous bands where they exist. In addition muscles must be brought back to their normal strength. The *first principle is to revascularise the area*. If a really acute hyperaemia can be produced some absorption of exudate not yet fully organised may occur. The tissues will be softened and relaxed and stretching made much easier. Revascularisation of a localised area may be produced in many ways. Sometimes an injection of a local anaesthetic may be used; this will overcome vaso-spasm by paralysis of vaso-constrictor fibres and so will promote a hyperaemia. An even greater effect may be obtained by following the injection by the application of really deep frictions. Deep massage alone will prove effective.

These measures are most successful in such conditions as chronic bursitis or chronic non-tubercular teno-synovitis, and fibrositis. Histamine or renotin ionisation or a strong dose of ultraviolet light can also be used to produce local hyperaemia, and are particularly effective if the thickened area is superficial, and a counter-irritant effect is desired.

Alternatively, some form of deep heating, such as ultra sound or short-wave diathermy, will be useful to increase the deep circulation.

The second principle is to follow the revascularisation by a deliberate attempt *to separate out, stretch and even break up the fibrous strands*. The best possible means of doing this is to use ultra sound or deep transverse frictions or, where suitable, vigorous active exercises.

If the chronic inflammation has resulted in muscle atrophy it is *essential to improve the condition of the muscle*. If muscles are in a very poor condition, faradism may be used to show the patient how to use his muscles, active contractions may then be combined with the faradism and very soon active work will replace electrical stimulation. Exercise may be quickly progressed and continued until the muscle condition equals that of the same group of the opposite limb.

SUPPURATIVE INFLAMMATION

It is well to remember that pus formation means destruction of tissue, and destroyed tissue must eventually be replaced, to a great extent at least, by scar tissue, with resultant alteration in function of the part. The great essential, therefore, where suppuration has occurred, is to limit as far as possible the production of pus and destruction of tissue, so that less fibrous tissue formation takes place.

The first principle of treatment, once the condition is established, is *to destroy micro-organisms and prevent their multiplication*. Destruction may be attempted by means of chemotherapy (that is the use of substances such as penicillin which destroy bacteria without devitalizing body tissues); by keeping septic surfaces clean; and by promoting free drainage of pus.

If pus is allowed to escape easily there will be less pressure in abscess cavities, less toxic absorption will take place and less destruction of tissue will occur. Destruction of bacteria and cleansing of surfaces may be aided by the use of short-wave therapy, ultra-violet rays and zinc ionisation. Once this principle has been fulfilled and free drainage is established, the next step is *to encourage rapid healing and to prevent contracture of fibrous tissue*. The promotion of a good blood supply will do much to promote rapid healing, and this can be aided by the use of infra-red or ultra-violet rays. Provided free drainage is present, circulation will be aided and fibrous contractures prevented by the use of small range, gentle, active movements, taking aseptic precautions in any necessary handling of the area.

Stiff joints are one of the complications of suppurative inflammation because circulation is impaired by the necessity for resting the part, and by the action of the toxins on the vessel walls. Oedema is also not an uncommon feature. A further principle of treatment is therefore *to prevent limited movement in joints*. Elevation of the part, and early active movements will relieve oedema and prevent joint stiffness. They can be commenced as soon as drainage is established. If the patient is being treated by saline baths the movements may well be carried out in the bath.

As in chronic inflammation, muscle atrophy is likely to be severe, and should be lessened by the measures taken to promote circulation and prevent stiff joints.

Later, when suppuration ceases, wounds are healed, and destroyed tissue has been replaced, massage may be used to soften and stretch fibrous tissue and loosen scars and keep them supple and free.

One principle applies to all types of inflammation—*the restoration of normal function*. Tissues may be pliable and elastic, joints may possess a full range of movement, perfect healing of ulcers and sinuses may have occurred and muscle tone and bulk may be normal, and yet the patient is unable to use his limb correctly. The lack may be partly mental, in that the patient is unable to realise that the part of the body is now organically sound. It is often due to a lack of co-ordination, the damaged structure not having learnt to fit in with healthy structures. This must be put right before the rehabilitation of the patient is considered complete.

OEDEMA

The treatment of oedema depends upon the type. General oedema is rarely treated by physical measures. In these cases the treatment is medical,

D

and if the heart lesion or the kidney disease can be alleviated oedema is likely to disappear. Occasionally a case of cardiac oedema is met with by the physiotherapist, when the main object is to hasten the absorption of fluid by the lymphatic vessels and so give the patient temporary relief from discomfort until such time as the production of excessive fluid ceases. This oedema will be treated on the same lines as obstructive oedema but with particular precautions owing to the cardiac condition.

Local oedema more commonly presents itself for physical treatment and a careful consideration of the type must first be made.

TRAUMATIC OEDEMA

If the trauma is extensive some oedema is almost inevitable. The main principle of treatment is, therefore, the prevention of organisation into fibrous tissue. Efforts must be made to decrease the formation of the tissue fluid, to speed its absorption and to keep it moving so that it cannot clot. Less fluid will be formed if rest and firm support are given. To increase the speed with which the fluid is absorbed it is necessary to encourage its movement into areas in which the veins and lymphatics have not been damaged and to speed the flow of venous blood and lymph in these regions. Such measures as superficial heat and massage to the region proximal to the injury will assist. Elevation of the limb is essential and, in this position rhythmic muscular contractions will press the fluid out of the tissue spaces. If these are difficult to obtain, minimal faradic contractions may be used temporarily. In nearly every case, functional use of the limb can be encouraged early, so stimulating the tissue drainage and preventing organisation.

OBSTRUCTIVE OEDEMA

The excess fluid in this case is the result of obstruction in the venous or lymphatic vessels, or in both. Whether or not the oedema will subside, depends upon how well the unobstructed vessels will dilate to do the work of the obstructed ones. The principle underlying the use of physical means is, therefore, the attempt to encourage the development of a good collateral circulation. Any measures which press the fluid out of the tissue spaces and force it proximally are likely to assist. Faradism under pressure, strong muscle contractions followed by relaxation, and kneadings given with deep pressure and relaxation are all effective. With the limb elevated, the fluid will be mechanically pushed on by slow, deep effleurage and vigorous active movements which press the fluid on in the veins and lymphatics. Regurgitation is prevented by the presence of valves.

A firm support should be applied to help to prevent accumulation of fluid. A one-way stretch elastic bandage must be worn and it is the physio-therapist's duty to teach the patient how and when to apply it and to give instructions about washing the bandage and its replacement when neces-sary.

In these cases of obstructive oedema the condition is sometimes a long-standing one and some of the tissue fluid may have organised into firm fibrous tissue which by pressure has further impeded the circulation. Special measures are then needed to soften this tissue. Any physical means which floods the tissue with blood and stretches it will be valuable; thus histamine or renotin ionisation and really deep massage may be used.

PARALYTIC OEDEMA

Since the excess fluid is the result of vaso-dilatation and lack of use, it is difficult to prevent its formation. Its continual dispersion and move-ment to prevent clotting are, therefore, essential. Unlike traumatic oedema this cannot be carried out by the use of rhythmic contractions and active movements. Passive means are therefore necessary. Elevation of the part is helpful. Artificial exercise of the paralysed muscles by means of the interrupted galvanic current will exert a pumping effect on the veins and lymphatics and will keep the tissue fluid moving. Passive movements of joints will have the same effect. Light massage is sometimes effective in dispersing the fluid into regions not affected by the paralysis, but care must be used not to increase the paralytic vaso-dilatation nor to bruise or stretch the atonic muscle fibres.

OEDEMA DUE TO POOR MUSCLE TONE
AND LAXITY OF THE FASCIA

Since the oedema is the result of lack of muscle tone and poor condition of fascia, the principle of treatment by physiotherapy is to bring back to normal the strength and tone of the musculature. This can be carried out by the use of maximal resisted exercises. During the time taken to bring the muscles and fascia back to normal, constant seeping of fluid into the tissues should be lessened by repeated elevation of the limb and by firm pressure in the form of Viscopaste or elastic bandages. Such fluid as does form must not be allowed to organise and measures such as those used in obstructive oedema are of value.

In all cases of oedema it is worth noting that the vessels in the region of the oedema should not be encouraged to dilate since this results in increased filtration. However, dilatation of vessels which are not always patent is desirable in areas proximal to the oedema. For this reason it is wiser to avoid the use of heat directly over the area. The immersion of an oede-matous hand or foot in hot paraffin wax usually increases the tension in the tissues. Similarly the use of hot baths is unwise. If these are used for the legs they also mean that the treatment is being carried out in the dependent position. If, as a result of oedema and arterial spasm, the limb is cold and blue, heat can be given to the trunk; the limb is then indirectly warmed without increasing the oedema.

PART II

Rheumatic Diseases

REVISED BY

JEAN WILHELM, M.C.S.P.

CHAPTER 1

Classification of Diseases in Rheumatology

THERE HAVE BEEN SEVERAL different classifications of rheumatic diseases and syndromes and these will probably be varied as knowledge increases. It is convenient at present to divide them into two main headings, Articular and Non-Articular, and then to sub-divide them further.

ARTICULAR

Known Aetiology

Infective	Staphylococcal	Tuberculous
	Gonococcal	Rubella
	Glandular fever	Mumps, etc.
Metabolic	Gout	
Degenerative	Osteo-arthrosis	Cervical spondylosis
Neuropathic	Syringomyelia	Diabetes mellitus

Uncertain Aetiology

Acute	Rheumatic fever	
Chronic	Rheumatoid arthritis and its variants:	
	Still's disease	Palindromic arthritis
	Felty's syndrome	Sjögren's syndrome
	Reiter's syndrome	Ankylosing spondylitis
	Psoriatic arthritis	Systemic lupus erythematosus
	Scleroderma	
Miscellaneous	Ulcerative colitis	

NON-ARTICULAR

Fibrositis	Myositis
Tendinitis	Tenosynovitis
Bursitis	Capsulitis

No attempt will be made in this brief section to describe in detail all the conditions set out in this classification. Acute rheumatic fever is not treated by physical means. Many years after the attack the physiotherapist may be asked to treat a patient suffering from congestive cardiac failure, the late result of the effect of acute rheumatism on the valves of the heart. The conditions most often reaching the Physiotherapy department—infective arthritis, gout, osteo-arthrosis, cervical spondylosis, rheumatoid arthritis, ankylosing spondylitis and non-articular rheumatism will be discussed here, and a few of the main points of the other conditions mentioned.

INFECTIVE ARTHRITIS

The gonococcus, pneumococcus and streptococcus are the organisms commonly responsible for infective arthritis. Streptococcal arthritis may follow streptococcal tonsillitis, while pneumococcal arthritis arises as a rule in association with pneumonia. In both streptococcal and pneumococcal arthritis, the exudate is usually purulent, while in gonococcal arthritis, which tends to follow in the wake of an attack of gonorrhoea, the effusion in the joint is sero-fibrinous. Whatever the causal organism, the arthritis may be monarticular or multiple joints may be involved. The knee is very commonly affected, particularly by gonorrhoea. Antibiotic therapy with penicillin or sulphanilamide drugs, usually brings about a speedy resolution of the arthritis, but the joints have a tendency to be left stiff and immobile, and in the prevention of this unfortunate legacy, the physiotherapist is often of great value. Abortus fever and bacillary dysentery sometimes produce a variety of infective arthritis which is very similar to rheumatoid arthritis.

Apart from antibiotic therapy, rest is the main principle of treatment of the joint or joints involved. Often a plaster splint is necessary, though it is sometimes bi-valved so that the condition of the joint can be watched. As soon as the acute symptoms have subsided, it is essential to prevent further muscle atrophy and to try to prevent organisation and adhesion formation within the joint and between the peri-articular structures. For this reason, assisted active movements within the limit of pain are essential, and rhythmic muscle contractions should be given repeatedly. The administration of deep heat is not wise while the condition is active since the metabolism and activity of the micro-organisms might be increased. Superficial heating for the relief of pain and relaxation of muscle spasm is safe and useful. Massage may help the condition of muscle groups but should not be used over the joint.

GOUT

Gout is a metabolic disorder in which purine metabolism is upset. The quantity of uric acid in the blood stream rises and from time to time there occurs a sudden precipitation of this substance into the tissues in the form of crystals of sodium biurate. These crystals are deposited in the cartilage, bone ends, synovial membrane and periarticular structures, and in addition, in other poorly vascularised structures such as the cartilage of the ears. These form the chalk stones or 'tophi' characteristic of gout.

During an acute attack of gout the deposit of sodium biurate in joint structure sets up an acute inflammatory reaction and the joint affected, commonly the metatarsophalangeal joint of the first toe, becomes red, hot, swollen and exquisitely painful and tender to touch, while over it the skin is stretched and shiny. When it occurs in larger joints such as the elbow or knee, the skin will not necessarily be very red, but it will be dry, whereas in many other forms of arthritis, the skin will be moist.

Such an attack lasts with varying degrees of intensity of pain over several days and then, as the joint symptoms subside, the skin desquamates. Usually the joint condition clears completely. If repeated attacks take place, arthritic changes will eventually occur and the joint will become stiff and the range of movement limited.

For such cases the treatment is purely medical. Colchicine or phenyl-butazone are the drugs in common use for suppressing an acute attack, but the patient may also be given Benemid, Anturan or other uricosurics to increase the excretion of urates through the kidneys: in course of time, tophi become re-absorbed.

Now that drugs play such an important part in controlling metabolism, diet is not as rigorous as it once was, but offal should in general be avoided, and also any food or drinks which the patients know will precipitate an acute attack.

Some patients suffer from a chronic form of gout in which acute attacks do not occur. For many weeks or months the patient complains of some pain, swelling and stiffness, usually in the small joints of the hands and feet, particularly the metatarsophalangeal joint of the great toe and similar joints in the fingers and thumb. Occasionally larger joints are also affected. Very often the joints fail to clear completely. In most cases tophi form, and, acting as irritants, result in degenerative osteo-arthritic changes. If the tophi form in superficial tissues the skin directly over them is so thin and shiny that they can be seen through it. Eventually, they tend to ulcerate through, necessitating surgical intervention to remove the tophi.

Again, the treatment is mainly medical, but physiotherapy is sometimes ordered to restore, maintain and increase the mobility of affected joints and atrophied muscles.

CHAPTER 2

Osteo-arthrosis. Cervical Spondylosis

OSTEO-ARTHROSIS IS A CONDITION affecting only the joints. The lesions are not disseminated in other tissues as in rheumatoid arthritis. Correlated with this is the fact that general constitutional symptoms are absent. In the majority of cases, osteo-arthrosis develops in the middle-aged and elderly and appears in those joints which are most subjected to strain: either the weight-bearing joints, such as the hip and knee, or those which, according to the particular occupation, are most used, such as the spinal articulations of the agricultural and manual worker, or the terminal interphalangeal joints of the hands of the gardener or cleaner.

Though much discussion exists as to the exact cause of the development of osteo-arthrosis, it is likely that the resistance of the joint structures is reduced by the 'wear and tear' of life. Minor traumata, sufficient to damage delicate joint structures, though insufficient to produce joint symptoms, may be responsible for the insidious onset of changes in cartilage and bone. Such stresses and strains may be seen in the osteo-arthrosis of certain definite occupations, as in the vertebral column of the miner and the elbow joint of the blacksmith.

Direct trauma, such as a fracture involving the articular surfaces and damaging the cartilage, is often followed by osteo-arthrosis. Faulty posture is a possible cause of degenerative changes because it upsets the mechanics of the joint, and abnormal strain is, therefore, brought to bear on cartilage and bone, as well as on joint capsules. For example, osteo-arthrosis of the spine is often secondary to structural kyphosis or scoliosis. Congenital abnormalities are liable to produce trouble in the same way. In many cases, early senile changes are probably the beginning of a chronic osteo-arthrosis.

Obesity is an important contributory factor in osteo-arthrosis of the hip, and knee, while varus or valgus deformity and repeated damage of the menisci are often followed by this type of arthritis in the knee joint.

PATHOLOGICAL CHANGES

These probably vary with the cause, the eventual condition of the joint being likely to be similar, whatever the cause.

If the changes are the result of wear and tear, they usually begin in the articular cartilage at the point at which trauma is applied. At first flakes of cartilage are desquamated from the surface and later fibrillation occurs, giving a velvety appearance. Erosion appears irregularly over the weight-bearing central zone and bony surfaces are exposed, these sclerose and become polished as a result of friction (eburnation).

In some cases the cartilaginous lesions take the form of irregular ulceration and proliferation, forming osteophytes of small size on the surface of the cartilage and they may become detached, forming a loose body.

Some time after the fibrillation of the central zone the cartilage at the periphery of the joint proliferates and irregular outgrowths occur, at first cartilaginous but later osseous. Initially they may take the form of lipping at the joint margin, but later the formation of long bony spurs or osteophytes, which may seriously interfere with movement (though ankylosis is rare) and locking may occur.

Heberden's nodes show in the fingers the proliferation of periosteum near the articular margin (see Plate I).

A third source of osteophyte formation is a fold of synovial membrane which becomes cartilaginous and then bony. This causes much difficulty in movement, and the peri-articular structures are eventually affected. Congestion or abnormal use will result in a hypertrophy of the synovial membrane with increased secretion of synovial fluid. Fringes and folds become enlarged and liable to be trapped on movement. The fibrosis of the capsule and ligaments resulting from continuous minor strain is followed by contracture, which, in its turn, will lead to limited movement and deformity.

SIGNS AND SYMPTOMS

In the early stages of the condition, there is usually hypotonia of the muscles acting on the affected joint, laxity of ligaments and a tendency for the joint to 'give way'. The range of movement is usually full, but the patient complains of pain at the extremes of each movement. There is also a feeling of stiffness on using the joint after a period of rest, and pain on weight-bearing or after prolonged exercise. As the degenerative changes progress, and fibrous thickening in the soft tissue develops, signs and symptoms become more pronounced. Pain and tenderness, enlargement of the joint, muscle atrophy, limitation of movement, deformity and crepitus are all common features.

Pain is a very variable feature and does not necessarily bear any relationship to the degree of cartilaginous or bony change, since the cartilage is devoid of nerve endings. According to its cause, it may be present at rest, particularly in bed when the limb becomes warm, or only on movement, or it may be persistent. It is most often felt after prolonged exercise or after a period of rest. It is usually experienced in the joint but may be referred. Referred pain occurs most often in osteo-arthrosis affecting the joints of the spine, since, as a result of changes in the joints between the articular processes, the intervertebral foramina may be narrowed and the spinal nerves compressed.

Pain may be the result of many different factors; nipping of the hypertrophied synovial membrane, fibrosis of the capsule or accessory ligaments, weakness and fatigue of muscles, or rubbing of 'young' osteophytes over one another.

Nipping of the hypertrophied synovial membrane gives rise to sharp pain and muscle spasm at one point of one particular movement. It ceases as soon as the fringe is released, leaving soreness and tenderness due to the inflammation which follows the trauma.

Fibrosis tends to cause trapping of nerve endings, so that when the contracting tissue is stretched, pain is felt. The pain is appreciated at that point in the range of movement which begins to stretch the contracted capsule or ligaments. As the disease progresses and contractures increase, pain is produced earlier in the movement. This may account for the onset of pain when the limb begins to get warm at night.

Tenderness is due either to inflammation of the synovial membrane which follows nipping, or to pressure on young osteophytes.

Joint enlargement. The swelling of an osteo-arthritic joint is often hard swelling. It is the result of an increase in the size of the bone ends by osteophyte formation, though it may also be partly due to fibrous thickening of the synovial membrane and capsule. Occasionally there will be an effusion into the joint. This will develop following trapping of the synovial membrane or minor strain of the joint.

Muscle weakness and atrophy. As pain and contractures develop, limited use and reflex inhibition lead to atrophy and weakness. The atrophy is rarely as obvious as it is in rheumatoid arthritis, and it is confined to the muscles acting on the joint.

Limited movement. At first, movement is limited only slightly when the shortened tissues are stretched. At this stage, the movement can often be completed passively if the patient will tolerate the discomfort. Later muscle weakness, spasm and contractures will limit both active and passive movements in all directions. When the joint space is lost and the cartilage is denuded, movement becomes mechanically difficult.

Deformity. This is a characteristic feature of the advanced condition. It may be the result of alteration of the alignment of the articular surfaces when part of the cartilage has been completely worn away. In the knee

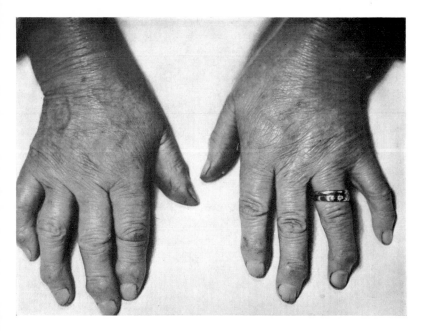

PLATE I. HEBERDEN'S NODES (*see pp.* 41 *and* 43)

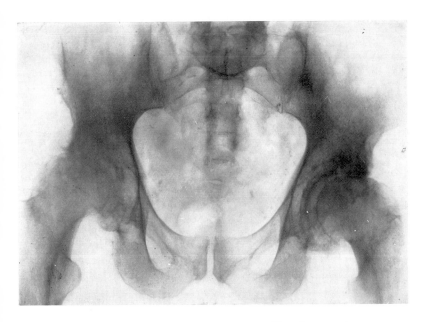

PLATE II. OSTEO-ARTHROSIS OF BOTH HIPS (*see p.* 41)

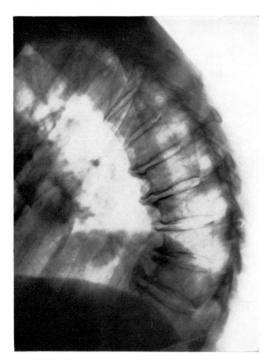

PLATE III (*see p.* 51)
(a) Showing lipping of the vertebrae at the anterior edge

(b) Osteo-arthrosis of the spine. Note the spurs of bone

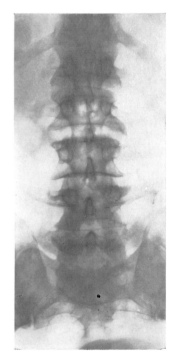

joint, for example, it may be only one condylar articulation which is affected and knock-knee may develop.

Deformity is also the result of thickening and contractures of the soft tissues, the direction depending upon which part of the capsule is most fibrosed. Thus at the hip joint the antero-lateral part of the capsule is usually eventually grossly thickened, and flexion and lateral rotation at the joint gradually develop.

Muscle imbalance will also predispose towards deformity, quadriceps weakness and hamstring spasm, leading to flexion deformity at the knee and abductor weakness and adductor spasm to adduction deformity at the hip. Spasm of a powerful muscle group will have a similar effect.

Often one deformity leads to another compensatory one; at the hip, for example, a flexion deformity, with increased pelvic tilt due to tight hip flexors, will result in a lordosis, and an adduction deformity will lead to a scoliosis, and the patient may stand with her knees flexed, with her foot resting on her toes.

A characteristic deformity of osteo-arthrosis results from the development of Heberden's nodes (Plate I). These may be either bony outgrowths, usually on the lateral side of the distal interphalangeal joints of the fingers, or small red cystic nodules containing gelatinous material. The former are often painless but unsightly, while the latter tend to develop suddenly and are then very painful.

Crepitus. In most osteo-arthritic joints, crepitus can be felt on movement. It usually occurs in joints in which there is irregular loss of cartilage and some bony outgrowths.

X-ray evidence. Changes can be seen in the X-ray photographs in advanced cases. The joint space is reduced. Sclerosis of the thin layer of compact tissue is appreciable. Bony outgrowths and cystic cavities are readily detectable. Too much emphasis should not, however, be laid on these findings since the actual bony changes do not necessarily tally with the degree of pain and loss of function.

Acute attacks. Occasionally osteo-arthrosis of a joint suddenly becomes acute. There is then swelling, intense pain, muscle spasm and very limited movement. This may follow minor strain, to which such joints are prone, or may be the result of trapping of some part of the hypertrophied synovial membrane.

PRINCIPLES OF TREATMENT BY PHYSIOTHERAPY

There are four fundamental objects of treatment in these cases; the first of these, and the most important to the patient, is relief of pain; the next three of equal importance are the relief of spasm and strengthening of muscles, the prevention of deformity and the maintenance or improvement of the range of movement.

Relief of pain. There is no known cure for the osteo-arthritic joint, there can only be relief of symptoms. Of these, pain is the most outstanding and worries the patient most, in advanced cases seriously interfering with daily activities and with sleep. The relief of pain is, therefore, of the utmost importance. Measures taken to fulfil this object depend upon the cause of pain. Analgesics, and sometimes injections of hydrocortisone into the joint, are given.

Should pain be due to fibrosis of the capsule and synovial membrane, heat may be successful, but in this case indirectly only, by softening the tissue so that it can be more readily stretched. Then the pain which occurs on movement, because soft tissue is being stretched, will occur less early. Heating should be followed by non-weight-bearing active exercises within the limit of pain. Occasionally, especially where there are cystic cavities in the bone, the application of heat increases the pain during its administration, and ice sometimes gives more relief, and is particularly useful in relieving spasm.

If nipping of a synovial fringe is causing pain, the avoidance of the particular movement will stop the irritation and the inflammation of the fringe may be relieved by intra-articular steroids.

Strengthening of muscles. This is necessary in all cases of osteo-arthrosis because the muscles are an essential support of the joint. Strong muscles will also be one factor in the prevention of deformity. All muscles acting on the joint should, therefore, be exercised in such a way as to increase their power and their endurance. Particular attention should be paid to those which will resist the tendency to the development of deformity. Thus at the hip, the extensors and abductors require special care. It will be borne in mind that three half-hour periods of exercise weekly will not achieve this object; it must be made certain that the patient practises repeatedly at home.

Prevention of deformity. The development of deformity at a joint will not only lead to increasing muscle weakness, to pain and to limited function, but also result in strain on other joints and compensatory deformities. For this reason deformities should, if possible, be avoided. The first essential is an understanding of the mechanics involved. Deformities will develop in the direction encouraged by the pull of the strong muscle groups and by contracture of the capsule. At the hip the tendency is for a flexion, adduction, lateral rotation deformity; at the knee, flexion and valgus; at the elbow, flexion.

The tendency is more easily checked before it has developed. The three most important measures are active assisted movements, active strengthening exercises, and the use of night splints. Active assisted movements are particularly valuable because in the early stages of the condition full range can be obtained, but often this is not done and consequently an insidious contracture develops.

Proprioceptive facilitation techniques are excellent both for assisting relaxation of inhibiting muscles and for building up the muscles necessary to resist deformity. Sling exercises are often helpful for osteo-arthritic hips, and patients do particularly well in the pool. Care must, however, be taken that they also have a repertoire of home exercises that they can do on dry land.

If contractures are responsible for limited movements, steps should be taken to stretch the soft tissue, followed by work to strengthen the muscles.

Occasionally a patient is seen in whom movement is so limited that there is little hope of increasing the range, in fact an arthrodesis is likely. These patients must be encouraged to develop a compensatory mechanism. A stiff hip is not so detrimental if the lumbar spine is reasonably mobile, so that adequate flexion is possible, and if the knee is more than normally mobile so that good flexion will allow the patient to put on her own shoes and stockings working from behind instead of in front.

Similarly a stiff knee will be helped by good range in the hip, and particularly in the ankle.

EXAMINATION OF THE PATIENT

This will follow lines similar to those described in a succeeding chapter for patients suffering from rheumatoid arthritis. Its purpose is to find out those things which make for suitable selection of treatment. Let us take for example the patient sent to the physiotherapy department ordered heat and exercises for an osteo-arthritic hip. It is essential to know whether there is pain and when it is felt, what is the state of the muscles, if there is any deformity and what is its cause if present, and how much limitation of movement there is. The first step, having read the notes and examined the X-rays, is to watch the patient as unobtrusively as possible as she walks into the department, noting how she walks, the presence of any limp and the facial expression. She is then observed as she undresses. Can she, for example, flex the hip to undo her shoes, and, if not, how does she manage?

Observation. Careful note is made of the position of the leg in lying. Are the hip and knee slightly flexed? If the pelvis is horizontal, what angle do the two legs make with the pelvis? Is the affected one adducted? Does one leg lie in greater lateral rotation than the other? The position of the lumbar spine is also noted. The gluteal muscles and the quadriceps are carefully observed, as these often show some atrophy. Comparison is made with the unaffected side.

Palpation. This is carried out to detect the presence of tenderness. Gentle pressure is given just below the middle of the inguinal ligament and around the great trochanter.

Measurements. The length of the leg is measured, since real or apparent shortening may be present. The bulk of the thigh and the degree of movement of the hip should be estimated.

Movements. Free active movements should be tested. Each movement is first carried out at the unaffected hip so that a careful comparison can be made. In the early stages the movement may be so little affected that, unless this is done, slight limitation is not detected. While the movements are being performed a close watch is kept for any movement of the pelvis and for the speed and smoothness of performance and signs of pain. Any movement which is even slightly limited is next tested passively and note is made as to what is the 'feel' of the limitation. Does it in fact feel like a bony block, or is there an elastic resistance, or is it muscle spasm due to pain?

If there appeared, during this observation, to be a flexion deformity, the opposite hip should be fully flexed and note made as to whether the affected leg increased in flexion during this test. Ability to correct this deformity may be tested by asking the patient to try to keep the affected leg on the bed while the unaffected hip is being flexed.

Slight limitation of adduction can best be checked by abducting both hips together. The mobility of the lumbar spine and knee should also be tested.

Power of muscles. Each group of muscles must be carefully checked by comparison with the unaffected hip using free and resisted movements, providing the latter are not painful. The abdominal muscles should be included in this test.

Posture. The patient is seen in the standing position and careful note is made of the position of the legs, pelvis and spine. With a marked adduction deformity the patient will attempt to bring the two legs parallel with one another by lifting the pelvis on the affected side, then to bring the foot on to the ground the knee on the unaffected side is flexed. If there is a hip flexion deformity, the pelvis will be tilted forward and there will be a marked lordosis and protruberant abdomen. If outward rotation of the hip has occurred, the patella will face laterally instead of directly forward, and the foot will be turned outwards.

Gait. The patient may walk with a characteristic dipping of the pelvis towards the leg that is off the ground (the Trendelenburg gait), and may require a stick. Should she need crutches, these will probably have been ordered by the physician, but the physiotherapist should make sure that sticks and crutches are the right length, and the patient is using them correctly. Her ability to mount steps, to get up and sit down, put on shoes and stockings should be tested and, if necessary, she can be given aids to help her.

ADVICE TO THE PATIENT

It should be emphasised that exercises three times weekly are of little value. Since exercises form, in most cases, the main part of the physical treatment, it is essential that they are practised daily, and if possible, several times daily. Each patient is given a written list of carefully chosen exercises with full instructions as to how, when and how often they should be done. The value of each exercise is explained, together with a little information as to what is likely to develop if they are not practised.

Instruction is also needed in relation to the amount of activity which should be undertaken. Usually this is done by the physician, but sometimes it is left to the physiotherapist. Exercise is absolutely essential if stiffness and limitation of movement is to be prevented. The patient is, therefore, instructed to carry on a normal, active life, and to learn her own limitations, how far she can walk without pain, to do her exercises always, using her full range of movement rather than lots of irritating small movements and to rest if an acute attack should occur. If the joints of the lower limb are affected, she should be advised not to stand more than is essential. A stool of suitable height will make it possible to sit while washing dishes, peeling potatoes and even ironing. Patients with osteo-arthrosis of the hip should spend some part of each day lying prone with feet wide apart to stretch the hip flexors and prevent the adductors from shortening further. She should also be told not to carry heavy shopping baskets.

If the patient is obese, she will probably have been told by the physician to lose weight and the physiotherapist can help by showing an interest and weighing her once a week.

If this advice is followed the patient can do a very great deal to make herself more comfortable and slow the progress of the disease.

SURGERY IN OSTEO-ARTHROSIS

As osteo-arthrosis is not a generalised disease, each joint can be dealt with separately as a mechanical problem in relation to the patient's symptoms, age and occupation.

THE HIP JOINT. The choice lies between arthrodesis, arthroplasty and osteotomy.

E

1. *Arthrodesis* is an operation, which, by fixing the joint, renders it pain free. It is used mainly for young people with one hip affected, because it requires good mobility of the lumbar spine and knee to compensate for a stiff hip.

Arthrodesis is also extremely successful in the knee, wrist, thumb, ankle and tarsal joints.

2. *Arthroplasty* is the construction of a new, movable joint. In practice, it is mainly confined to the elbow, the hip, metacarpophalangeal and metatarsophalangeal joints. There are three main types of arthroplasty.

A. *Excision arthroplasty* (Girdlestone pseudarthrosis) in which one or both ends of the bones are excised. The gap fills with fibrous tissue, or a pad of muscle or soft tissue may be sewn in between the bones. This allows an increased range of movement, so that a patient may, for instance, sit more comfortably, but the joint lacks stability unless the muscles surrounding it are strong enough to support it.

B. *Cup arthroplasty* is virtually limited to the hip joint. The joint surfaces are refashioned and a cup, usually vitallium, is inserted over the head of the femur. This method allows good mobility and is sometimes used in conjunction with an arthrodesis of the other hip.

C. *Replacement arthroplasty*. One or both of the articulating bone ends is excised and replaced by a metal prosthesis. There are several methods, notably Judet and Austin Moore.

3. *Osteotomy* (McMurray displacement osteotomy). The femur is divided at the level of the lower margin of the acetabulum and the shaft fragment displaced medially to lie close under the acetabulum. The fragments are secured in the new position and weight is transmitted more directly through the pelvis to the femoral shaft and mechanical strain reduced.

THE KNEE JOINT. The patella is excised when severe patello-femoral arthrosis is evident, with pain, crepitus and difficulty in going downstairs as well as walking. If untreated, osteo-arthrosis affects the tibio-femoral joint.

Physiotherapy aims at strengthening muscles, improving mobility and re-educating the patient in walking, standing up and sitting down, and using stairs. This can best be done while in bed by static contractions to all muscles around the affected joint, and free active movements to all other joints, as far as possible. The exercises should be gradually progressed and the patient encouraged to be as mobile as possible in bed. Exercises in the pool, partial weight-bearing and walking in the pool is an excellent way to give the patient confidence. 'Skates' on a large piece of hardboard can be used to increase the range of abduction of the hip. Later slings and springs are valuable and the patient can graduate from crutches to sticks.

CERVICAL SPONDYLOSIS

Recurring attacks of pain in the neck and arm are most frequently caused by cervical spondylosis.

The apophyseal joints of the spine are synovial and therefore susceptible to the same pathological processes which involve synovial joints elsewhere. They may thus be the site of a primary osteo-arthrosis, or of a secondary osteo-arthrosis due to the degeneration of the intervertebral disc and consequent narrowing of the disc space, or a lesion of the vertebrae or ligaments, and it is usually impossible to be certain to what extent the symptoms are due to the osteo-arthrosis or to the associated lesion.

Cervical spondylosis is more common in women than in men, and occurs mainly from middle age onwards.

It is important to note that degeneration and proliferation of bone take place in very close proximity to the intervertebral foramina, and a large osteophyte, or slight alteration in the alignment of the articular surfaces, or a degenerated disc, may bring about narrowing of a foramen, and therefore compression of a sensory nerve root, producing pins and needles, numbness or pain. If a foramen is narrowed it may still be large enough not to press on a nerve root at rest, but on certain movements pressure may be exerted. In this case nerve root pain is intermittent. Thickening of the capsule and periarticular structures may also result in pressure on a nerve root.

Pain and limited movement are the chief features of cervical spondylosis. Pain is present on movement, is relieved by rest, but is worse on moving after a period of rest. It can keep patients from sleeping at night, and they often find they are in more pain than they were during the day. The pain may be felt in the neck; over the occiput, sometimes producing headaches; in the shoulder girdle, radiating down the arm; and in the upper anterior chest if the disc between the 7th cervical and 1st thoracic vertebrae is affected. Both passive and active movements are limited by muscle spasm. In the acute stage the patient may be in bed, having analgesics and possibly continuous traction. She may also be provided with a collar.

TREATMENT BY PHYSIOTHERAPY

Heat, shortwave diathermy or hot pads and sometimes massage, are given to relax the muscles and relieve pain, preparatory to mobilising the neck or giving traction.

Mobilisation. All free movements of the head, neck and shoulders should be taught, and the patient encouraged to do exercises at home several times a day. If the patient is in great pain head rotation can be given in lying, and hold relax techniques used to encourage relaxation as many patients are of an anxious disposition and tend to tense their shoulder muscles. Mobilising techniques can be very helpful.

Advice should be given as to the ordinary things of life; not carrying heavy shopping bags or brief-cases, or lifting heavy weights; altering one's work position, having a chair of the right height and a good light to work by; and proper pillow support at night; all small things that can make a great difference.

Traction. Pressure is relieved if the vertebrae are separated, and root pain can sometimes be completely relieved if traction is properly applied. It can be given in several ways, either straight with the patient lying flat, or on an inclined plane; or in sitting; or traction in flexion.

In straight traction weights of about 7 lb. are used, and the weights gradually increased until root signs have disappeared, usually at 10 to 14 lb. This is maintained for about 10 minutes providing the patient has no increase in pain or side-effects. Obviously times and weights will vary with the age and condition of the patient, and it may be necessary to go up to 20 lb. with a tough man.

Traction in flexion is most useful when the lower cervical vertebrae are affected and where there is root pain.

The patient lies flat with the head suspended in flexion by a weight of 10 to 14 lb. The physiotherapist should then try to find a pain-free position. The head may have to be rotated, and sometimes side-flexed slightly as well as flexed. Once the correct position is found the patient's head can be supported on pillows, and she should be encouraged to remain in that position for 15 minutes or longer. It should be explained to her that she may also get relief if she adopts the same position when going to bed at night.

Collars are frequently ordered and are very successful as a rule in correcting posture and relieving pain. They can be made of Plastazote, felt, Molefoam, Sorbo-rubber or plastic.

LIPPING OF THE VERTEBRAE AND THINNING OF THE DISC IN THE THORACIC AND LUMBAR SPINES

It is not uncommon to find that after a period of years degenerative changes develop in the intervertebral disc which becomes considerably thinned. The nucleus pulposus becomes smaller and easily herniates. The buffering effect of the disc is then lost and pressure on movement is no longer distributed evenly over the surface of the vertebrae. The front of the body is therefore subjected to greatest strain and it tends to respond by throwing out extra bone (see Plate IIIA). Sometimes the annulus fibrosus may become so thin that the edges of the vertebrae actually come into contact on movement and irritation also results in bony proliferation. Bony spurs are formed (see Plate IIIB) and occasionally these may fuse, bridging across the gap between two vertebrae. There is sometimes an involvement of the articular joints, with the changes of true osteo-arthrosis, when the disc changes have developed, since the thinning of the disc may lead to altered alignment and persistent strain on these joints.

Quite often the patient is free from symptoms, but sometimes there is the gradual onset of stiffness and aching in the affected region of the back. Occasionally nerve roots may be involved, since much narrowing of the disc space will reduce the size of the intervertebral foramen.

TREATMENT BY PHYSIOTHERAPY

As with the other inflamed joints, rest is all-important in the acute stage, particularly if there is root pain present. The patient should rest in bed on a firm mattress or preferably with a piece of hardboard under the mattress until the very acute stage has passed.

When the pain lessens, some form of heat, either infra-red or short wave diathermy, followed by abdominal exercises, extension exercises for the back, and re-training in posture should be given. The patient should also be taught the best ways to pick up things from the floor, to lift, to carry bags, to make beds, etc.

Should the patient be obese, she will probably have been told to lose weight, and it will be a great help to her if the physiotherapist weighs her regularly.

Lumbar traction is also sometimes given, particularly if there is root pain. If these treatments fail to give relief, the patient is generally prescribed a surgical corset.

CHAPTER 3

Rheumatoid Arthritis and its Variants. The Diffuse Collagen Diseases

IN ITS 'PRIMER' on this subject the Expert Committee on Chronic Rheumatic Diseases appointed by the World Health Organisation (1954) included the 'Collagen group' of diseases in their classification of 'pararheumatic' disease.

Collagen forms the bulk of connective tissue and the three elements, cellular, fibrillary and ground tissue, are closely associated with the skin, blood and lymph vessels, nerves and visceral organs, all of which may be affected. The collagen diseases are grouped together because (i) they have many symptoms in common and many overlap, (ii) they show an immunological abnormality and (iii) because of the fundamental part played by intercellular substances in these conditions. It has been suggested that auto-immunity (the production of antibodies against a constituent of the individual's own body) may result in connective tissue disease. But virus and bacterial infections have not been excluded and research continues. The main diseases grouped under this heading are:

rheumatoid arthritis, systemic lupus erythematosus, polyarteritis nodosa, scleroderma, dermatomyositis, cranial arteritis, Sjögren's syndrome.

RHEUMATOID ARTHRITIS

This is a subacute or chronic, non-suppurative inflammatory polyarthritis affecting mainly the peripheral joints, usually symmetrical, running a prolonged course of exacerbation and remission, accompanied by signs of a systemic disturbance such as anaemia, weight loss and a raised erythrocyte sedimentation rate.

The onset is most common between the ages of forty and sixty, though no age group is exempt; it attacks women more often than men. In a small percentage the disease comes on suddenly with an acute febrile illness; in the great majority of cases the onset is insidious. The symptoms are those of pain and stiffness. Often at this stage there may be no objective evidence

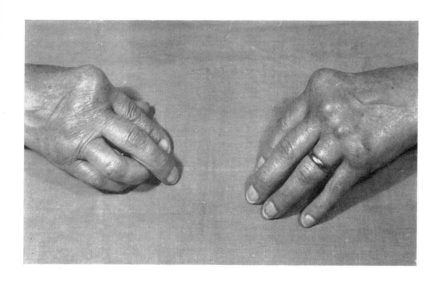

PLATE IV. RHEUMATOID ARTHRITIS (*see p.* 53)
(a) Showing deformity of hands

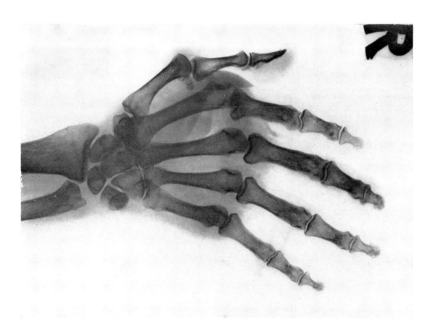

(b) X-ray photograph of same patient

PLATE V. (*See p.* 56). Showing typical attrition rupture of the extensor tendons due to rheumatoid involvement of the inferior radio-ulnar joint. The lower end of the ulna is subluxated in both hands.

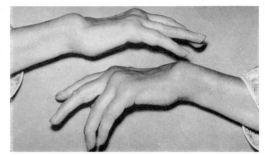

PLATE VI. (*See p.* 59). Attrition rupture of extensor tendons to the ring and little fingers at the wrist. The probe points to spicules of bone arising from the lower end of the ulna. The tendons and disorganised rheumatoid granulation tissue are clearly seen. Behind the probe are the intact extensor tendons of the index and middle fingers.

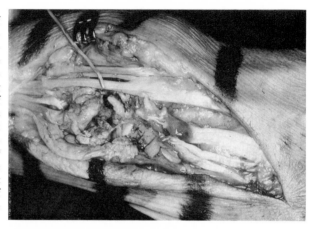

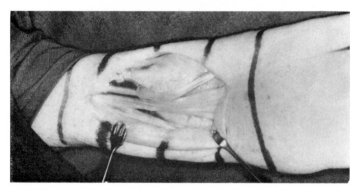

PLATE VII. (*See p.* 59). The lower end of the ulna is subluxated dorsally. No attrition of the extensor tendons has yet occurred but the distorted paths and early rheumatoid infiltration is well shown. This patient if untreated would develop rupture of these extensor tendons.

of the disease process—either radiologically or in the erythrocyte sedimentation rate. Gradual swelling, deformity and restriction of movement develop. The small joints of the body are most commonly involved at first. Often the proximal interphalangeal joints of the fingers are first attacked. Gradually the disease involves the metacarpophalangeal and wrist joints (see Plate IV) and later the elbow and shoulder. Similarly the joints of the lower extremity are involved. The temporomandibular joints and joints of the cervical spine are also sometimes affected. The sacro-iliac joints and joints of the thoracic and lumbar spine are rarely attacked. The condition is usually bilateral, though occasionally asymmetrical.

There is no known cause for the disease. Heredity is thought to play a part, climate, housing and working conditions affect the arthritic and some observers believe that persons of a certain type of psychological make-up are more prone to develop the disease than others. Metabolic and endocrine disturbances can be associated with rheumatoid arthritis and it is an interesting fact that during pregnancy or jaundice, arthritic symptoms remit. It appears to be a disease of civilised people.

EXAMINATION OF THE PATIENT

Before the physiotherapist can treat the patient a careful examination is necessary. This examination fulfils a special purpose and is only partly similar to that carried out by the physician.

The purpose of the examination is three-fold. First, its purpose is to find out something of the patient's background, without which an assessment of suitable treatment cannot be made. Secondly, it is essential to know the state of the general health, how much work the patient is capable of, and what medical treatment she is having. Thirdly, it is necessary to have a knowledge of the present state of each affected joint. This changes so frequently that it is possible that the joint may not be in the same state when the patient reaches the department as it was when the patient was seen by the physician. The actual physical examination is always preceded by a thoughtful reading of the patient's notes. These will nearly always give the facts about the patient's general health, the level of the erythrocyte sedimentation rate, and the condition of the blood. Also in the notes will usually be found the social history of the patient, including such points as the number and age of the family, type of house, and the amount of help in the house. A detailed account of the state of the joints at the time of examination will also be included. It might well be asked what more do we need to know. The answer is not, in fact, difficult to seek. We must add, in order to carry out adequate and safe treatment, the state of the skin which tells us whether certain physical measures are suitable; the power of the muscle groups which guides us as to the most suitable type of exercise; the presence of pain, including how and when pain is produced; the degree of tenderness and its site, both of which help us in the placing of pads and electrodes and in the use or omission of massage and exercises. It is also necessary to know the degree of deformity, and if movement is limited, the reason for this limitation in terms of spasm, contracture or ankylosis. Perhaps most important of all, we have to ask: is the patient independent, what can she not do for herself?

No assessment of the needs of the patient from the point of view of physiotherapy can be made without first carrying out such an examination. Especially is this so when the physician, having gained confidence in the physiotherapist, orders 'physiotherapy.'

Method of examination

The first step in any examination is the study of the notes written by the physician. In most hospitals, these are readily available. In some cases the X-ray photographs and report will also give useful information.

The second step is the observation and questioning of the patient. The patient should, as far as is possible, be left to undress and settle down by herself, careful watch being kept to note her particular difficulties. When she is comfortably settled, warm and in a good light, her co-operation is obtained by an explanation of the purpose and method of the examination.

While talking to her, her general appearance will be noted. It is possible to begin to assess how depressed, how tense, how ill she may be, and how painful her joints are, and whether pain keeps her awake at night. A slight idea of the general muscular condition and posture and what joints are affected may also be obtained.

As the main aim of physiotherapy is to return the patient to a full normal life, or to assist her in overcoming her difficulties and making the fullest use of what powers remain with her, a very careful and detailed examination must be made, with particular attention being paid to the patient's ability to cope with the ordinary, but vital, things of daily life; such as the ability to get in and out of the bath, to wash the back of her neck and do her hair, to sit down on a lavatory seat, to turn a door handle and even to feed herself. An assessment chart is valuable.

The joints must not only be tested individually, but also as a functionally useful limb. The hand and arm are of paramount importance and will, therefore, be taken as an illustration.

The patient should be sufficiently undressed for both arms, shoulders and her neck to be seen easily, and also so that her movements are not impeded by clothes. In dealing with a rheumatoid patient, the hands should be examined carefully as the disease very often shows itself first in the hands and feet. The appearance and range of movement of the fingers, thumbs and wrists, the tenderness on pressure of individual joints and the strength of the patient's grip should be noted.

This is followed by testing the range and power of movement of the elbows and observing any painful spots such as occur in tennis elbow. The shoulders and acromio-clavicular joint should be put through the full range of all movements, or as much as the patient can manage, *both* actively and passively. Palpation of the shoulders will elicit any tender spots, and possibly crepitus will be felt. No examination of the shoulder would be complete without all the movements of the neck being tested also, as pain arising in the cervical region may sometimes be felt most intensely in the arm.

The patient should be watched during the whole procedure, because in spite of explanation, some patients will not readily admit to pain. Note is, therefore, made of muscle contraction, wincing and facial expression. One of the objects of these tests is to find out what particular change is leading to limited movement. If there is no movement at all, it is likely to be because there is bony ankylosis, or severe muscle spasm. Very slight movement is often the result of complete loss of cartilage and fibrous ankylosis. Some limitation is often present due to habit spasm or contractures. All movements should be kept within the limit of pain.

This could be followed by detailed examination of legs and spine.

From this examination it should be possible to decide the most useful form of physiotherapy and whether the patient needs any aids such as long-handled combs for doing her hair or thick-handled cutlery for feeding herself.

The third step is the careful examination of each individual joint. To make this clear, the knee joint will be taken as an illustration, but the same procedure may be used for any joint. The patient should be in the lying position with the head and shoulders comfortably raised, and no pillow should be used beneath the legs.

Observation. The legs should be viewed together and equally. A careful check of bulk of the quadriceps muscle, the position of the knee, the contour of the joint, the presence of swelling should be made. The knees are compared since there is rarely symmetry in this disease. Note may also be made of any movements the patient makes, because if the knees are painful, she often cannot keep them still for long.

Palpation. The swollen area should be gently palpated with the finger-tips to ascertain whether it feels soft, spongy or firm. If fluid is suspected, the flat hand may be gently placed above the supra-patellar pouch and pressure exerted towards the toes. If there is effusion the fluid will move and the patella will be floated off the lower end of the femur. Gentle pressure by the fingers of the free hand will cause the patella to tap against the femur. This tap can be felt.

Palpation is then carried out to note the presence or absence of tenderness and whether the tenderness is the result of 'activity' within the joint or a localised tenderness of ligaments or tendons. The joint is gently grasped between the hands and they are then gradually approximated, careful note being made of how much depth of pressure is required *before* pain is experienced. The patient is watched during this procedure. With the fingertips, palpation is carried out along the joint line, over the medial ligament, the ligamentum patellae and the insertions of the hamstrings.

Some knowledge of the state of the muscles may be gained by palpation. Tone can be tested by touch; the muscles vary in softness or firmness according to their state of tone.

Measurements. These are useful if there is any doubt as to difference in size, and for record purposes, to check the progress of the joint. The bulk of both thighs, circumference of the joint and the degree of flexion and extension should all be measured.

CHANGES IN THE JOINTS (See Plates V, VI and VII)

Changes in the joints often, though not always, progress through three stages.

Stage I. The synovial membrane becomes inflamed and is, therefore, hyperaemic and infiltrated by inflammatory cells. The secreting cells become more active and the result is an oedematous membrane and effusion into the joint cavity. Inflammation tends to spread, to involve the peri-articular soft tissues, the capsule, ligaments, bursae, tendons and their sheaths. Clinical examination shows a tender swollen joint with movement probably limited by pain and muscle spasm. If the disease is arrested at this stage, the joint can return to *normal* though there is no certainty that the inflammation will not flare up again at a later date.

Stage II. If the disease progresses, granulation tissue is formed within the synovial membrane and peri-articular structures. It tends to spread from the membrane over the periphery of the articular cartilage. The cartilage, now covered by this tissue, gradually thins and disintegrates, leaving areas of bone covered only by granulation. Sometimes granulation tissue invades the bone ends from the remains of the perichondrium and from the tissue growing in over the cartilage. Much decalcification of bone occurs, probably due to the hyperaemic condition around the bone ends.

With the destruction of articular cartilage and filling of the joint with granulation tissue, adhesions are formed between the synovial membrane and the thickened capsule and the tendons and their sheaths. Thus the joint movement is permanently impaired. Some cases never progress beyond the second stage and may retain a useful, though reduced, movement even in the face of active inflammation.

Stage III. The granulation tissue becomes organised into fibrous tissue and thus the soft tissues are matted together with adhesions forming between tendons and capsule and between the articular surfaces. Contractures develop and deformity and gross limitation of movement result. In such joints the articular surfaces may be partly covered with cartilage and partly with fibrous tissue, giving rise to much irregularity, or they may be completely joined by fibrous tissue or even by bone. Where such changes have occurred, little improvement in function can be expected.

ARTICULAR SIGNS AND SYMPTOMS

Joints in which some or all of these changes have developed will show certain characteristic features. Pain and tenderness, swelling, limitation of movement, muscle atrophy and deformity are all to be expected, though they will occur in differing degrees according to the severity of the changes.

Pain is present in all three stages.

In the first stage it is often continuous, and since several joints may be affected, the patient's life may be a misery unless the pain is medically controlled. Movement increases the pain, hence the joints tend to be held rigid. In the second stage, pain is often less noticeable at rest but is more marked on movement or weight-bearing, so that if the knees or ankles are involved, walking is a real difficulty. In the third stage, when inflammation has subsided and fibrous tissue has formed, there is usually no pain at rest but only on movement when the fibrous tissue is stretched and a pull is, therefore, exerted on sensitive tissues.

Tenderness will always be present when there is any active inflammation in the joint. It can be elicited by gentle pressure of the joint and by palpation along the joint line. The degree of tenderness is a good indication of the activity of the arthritis. When the inflammation has subsided there may still be tenderness, but this is localised and not on pressure of the joint. It is felt over structures which are being persistently irritated by stretching, the result of abnormal posture. For example, at the knee there is often localised tenderness over the ligamentum patellae, the tibial attachment of the medial ligament, and the insertion of the hamstrings. In the latter case, the tenderness may be explained by the fact that the hamstrings are often contracted and then pull on the periosteum at their insertions.

Swelling is usually present at all stages of the disease. In the stage of early inflammation, the swelling is soft, and often fluctuating owing to the presence of effusion. Sometimes there is oedema not limited to the joint only; for example, the whole finger or fingers and hand may be puffy, while if the joints of the lower extremity are affected, there is often oedema of the feet and legs. Later, as granulation tissue forms, the swelling feels firmer and more spongy. It is often at this stage more noticeable owing to muscle atrophy proximal and distal to the joint giving rise to the spindle-shaped or fusiform swelling so often described in textbooks.

Muscle spasm is a common feature. In the first stage the spasm is protective, its object being to prevent movement of a painful joint.

Muscle atrophy is an outstanding feature and is largely the result of disuse. If movement causes pain then the patient moves the joint as little as possible. In some patients, atrophy exceeds that which could be explained by disuse alone. Atrophy is a serious feature because it means less protection of the already damaged joint and more likelihood of the development of fixed deformity.

Deformity is one of the greatest dangers to fight against in rheumatoid arthritis. Each damaged joint has a characteristic deformity pattern. There is some position in which the capsule and ligaments are most relaxed and there is, therefore, most room for swelling with minimal pressure on nerve endings. In addition, at each joint, some muscle groups are more powerful than others. In many cases gravity has a powerful influence over the direction of the deformity. Thus we find a flexed knee, a dorsi-flexed everted ankle, clawed toes, adducted and medially rotated shoulder, flexed elbow, pronated forearm and flexed wrist. At the hand the deformity consists of ulnar deviation of the fingers, flexion of the metacarpophalangeal joints, hyper-extension of the proximal interphalangeal joints and adduction of the thumb. At first the deformities are held by muscle spasm, but later they become more fixed due to contracture of the muscle framework, permanent shortening of the muscle fibres and shortening of the fascia and ligaments. Later destructive changes predominate with subluxation and dislocation sometimes proceeding to fibrous or bony ankylosis.

Limited movement is another serious feature of the disease. In cases of gradual onset there is often a history of stiffness first thing in the morning which wears off during the day, but recurs after exercise and at night. If an acute attack develops, the joint movement becomes grossly limited by spasm. Later, movement is restricted in all directions as a result of muscle weakness and contractures, and, sometimes, because of gross destruction of the articular surfaces. Eventually, in some cases, movement is completely lost, due to fibrous or bony ankylosis.

It will be realised that no two cases are alike, and that each case varies from time to time. Thus there may be one joint at Stage I, another in Stage II, and several in the third stage, all at the same time. A joint in Stage III or Stage II may suddenly flare up and show all the features of acute inflammation. The disease is in fact unpredictable.

CHANGES IN OTHER TISSUES

As rheumatoid arthritis is one of the collagen diseases, other systems of the body may also become involved.

The skin is shiny, perspires freely, and becomes atrophic. A common feature is the formation of subcutaneous nodules around bony points, particularly around the elbow and along the posterior border of the ulna. These nodules have been found to consist of a central area of necrotic tissue, a group of phagocytic cells and an outer ring of proliferating connective tissue.

Muscles. Similar nodules form in the connective tissue framework of the muscles, and there is usually atrophy of the muscle fibres. Thus there is a general reduction in muscle bulk throughout the body predisposing to faulty posture and defective function. In later stages, there may be rupture of the extensor tendons (see Plates VI and VII), due to invasion of granulation tissue from the joint, or from erosion due to roughened bone ends at the wrist.

Lymphatic glands often show enlargement. The spleen is occasionally enlarged and the epitrochlear gland can be readily palpated at the elbow.

Vascular system. Patients often complain of cold hands and feet. This is due to vasoconstrictor spasm particularly in cold weather, although the occurrence of a diffuse inflammatory vasculitis has long been recognized in rheumatoid arthritis.

In general, during a fairly active phase of the disease, the patient presents, in addition to joint troubles, a picture of ill-health. Continuous pain leads to a sense of frustration, marked depression develops as the patient finds she cannot play her part in family life, and the worries and problems of life are liable to give her a 'flare-up' of the disease. There is a loss of weight and appetite, a feeling of lassitude bordering on exhaustion, and often anaemia and osteoporosis. The rheumatoid serum factor (Rose-Waaler test) is positive in eighty per cent of cases of over one year's duration and the erythrocyte sedimentation rate is raised.

PROGNOSIS

There is no known cure for the disease, but it is known that it sometimes eventually burns itself out. It is impossible to make a definite prognosis in the early stages of any case, though, in general, males do better than females, and patients who have the disease in a mild and limited form progress better than those with marked activity and extensive involvement. Patients brought into hospital for treatment within one year of onset of symptoms are most likely to do well, but it is a variable and fluctuant disease with periods of relapse and remission. In about twenty-five per cent of patients, the disease burns itself out within a year or two, leaving no crippling or deformity. In ten per cent the disease progresses inexorably in spite of all treatment, eventually leaving the patient a bed-ridden cripple. In the remaining sixty-five per cent of cases, the disease follows a course of exacerbations and remissions until it finally burns itself out after perhaps ten or twenty years. There is hope for this large group because, with proper care and their own co-operation, they can usually be kept ambulant and able to lead useful lives.

PRINCIPLES OF TREATMENT

In spite of continuous research, no cure has yet been found for the disease; treatment therefore has three main objects: improvement of health and so of the ability of the patient to fight the disease; relief of symptoms; maintenance of function of the joints.

Improvement of health. The first principle is *rest*. During an active phase of the disease when one or more joints are acutely inflamed and the general health is particularly poor, the patient should have complete rest in bed. She is often admitted to hospital in order to prevent her from doing household tasks, and to be helped perhaps by seeing others who are bearing and coping with disabilities greater than her own. Unless weight-bearing joints are acutely affected, the patient is usually allowed to get up for toilet purposes, and later for longer periods during the day. This type of rest, however, can never be satisfactory if the patient is tense because of social or financial worries and here the medical social worker may be able to help. Some relief from tension can be gained by training in relaxation and by the practice of breathing exercises. Good food, easily digested, and containing adequate first-class protein, vitamins and calcium are helpful, and iron is given to the patient if she is anaemic.

Relief of symptoms. The symptom which worries the patient above all is persistent pain, hampering activity, reducing sleep and so lowering general health and morale. Relief of pain is therefore an important principle as pain, if persistent, lowers the morale which in turn lowers the pain threshold.

Every effort is made to control the disease and the patient's pain with rest, simple analgesics and physical means, such as splinting, heat, massage and exercises, since all other methods have their dangers or side-effects. The physiotherapist should have some knowledge of these since she is often the first person to see or be told of discomfort or skin rashes, etc.

DRUGS AND THEIR SIDE-EFFECTS

Aspirin group. These are still the safest and most widely used analgesics in the early stages of the disease. Later they can be used in conjunction with steroids or gold. They are not drugs of addiction and the patient should be encouraged to take the number of tablets per day that the physician has ordered, since it is held that as the disease is incurable and often does not burn itself out for many years, the patient should not suffer unnecessary pain. The aspirin group produces few side-effects and is thought to be anti-inflammatory. The commonest side-effects of aspirin are dyspepsia and gastro-intestinal bleedings.

Phenylbutazone (Butazolidin) suppresses pain, but may produce dyspepsia leading to gastro-intestinal ulcers. For this reason it should be taken in the middle of a meal and not on an empty stomach, and the dose recommended by the physician should never be exceeded. Phenylbutazone can also produce nausea, skin rashes and fluid retention.

Gold is used chiefly in the active stage of rheumatoid arthritis where it may be effective in arresting the active progress of the disease. It is given, usually at weekly intervals, by intramuscular injections. The commonest side-effects are skin rashes, diarrhoea, stomatitis and albuminuria. It is important to look out for these symptoms during treatment and for some time after and report them. Liver and bone marrow damage can also occur. If ultra-violet light is being given, it should be remembered that gold is a sensitiser and doses should be reduced.

The anti-malarial drugs. Chloroquine and Plaquenil are sometimes used as an alternative to gold. The side-effects are nausea, giddiness, vomiting, diarrhoea, dermatitis, blurring of vision, corneal opacities and retinal derangement with pigmentation, which the patient sometimes reports as 'having bother with my eyes lately'.

Cortico-steroids are the most dangerous of the antirheumatoid drugs, and are not used unless the benefits that are likely to accrue are worth the hazards.

The most commonly employed are the oral preparations, prednisone and prednisolone. In larger doses they modify tissue reaction in pathological stages, but in rheumatoid arthritis, the maintenance dose suppresses the inflammatory reaction and is kept as small as possible, compatible with the degree of the patient's pain, because of the danger of side-effects.

When steroids are first given the patient feels so much better that the tendency is to overwork damaged joints. This is the 'honeymoon' period.

Once on steroids, withdrawal is difficult and the patient has to be weaned very slowly because her adrenals are not functioning. For this reason patients must never run out of their supply of tablets, and should always carry a steroid card indicating what treatment they are having. Surgery takes place under an 'umbrella' of increased steroid dose.

The possible side-effects of these preparations are:

1. Obesity, mooning of the face, sodium and fluid retention, muscle weakness, diabetes, osteoporosis (sometimes with fractures of the long bones and collapse of the vertebral bodies), hypertension, adrenal failure and emotional disturbances due to an exaggeration of the normal physiological action of the steroids.

2. The incidence of infection is not significantly increased, but when it occurs the symptoms may be suppressed and the patient may fail to report them. Healed or quiescent tubercular lesions may become active during treatment. Care must be taken to inform the doctor of any new signs or symptoms.

3. Dyspepsia and peptic ulceration; therefore steroids should always be taken with a meal.

Hydrocortisone or one of its derivatives is also used for topical application and for injection into painful areas, such as carpal tunnel or tennis elbow and joints. When it is used in this way to allay inflammation it has none of the side-effects mentioned above, though sometimes the joint is painful for some hours after the injection.

THE PART PLAYED BY PHYSIOTHERAPY

Pain, swelling and muscle spasm may also be relieved by the use of splints, heat, and in some cases, suitable movements. While it is not possible to prevent changes, it is possible to limit them and it is clearly essential to limit crippling and to help the patient to develop the patience, courage and perseverance necessary to fight the disease.

The general health. As has already been seen, bed rest is, in many cases, necessary. This has certain disadvantages. Circulation is slowed, general muscle atrophy develops, breathing is restricted and joints tend to become stiff. Good posture is difficult to maintain. Often the mattress sags, the pillows are unsuitably arranged, and the bedclothes are heavy on the feet. The result is that the head is pressed forward, the shoulders rounded, the chest narrowed and the lumbar curve obliterated. The knees may be flexed and the feet plantar flexed and everted. The patient, unchecked, tends to hold the arms in to the side, with the forearms resting across the abdomen, and, consequently, the fingers and wrists are flexed. All these disadvantages can be, at least, reduced by the use of physical measures. Slowing of the circulation and generalised muscle atrophy due to disuse may be dealt with by the use of easy movements. Each muscle group and each joint, excluding those which are acute or subacute, should be given free, simple movements using the full range of movement or as much of it as the patient is fit enough to do. Static exercises should be given to muscles controlling actively inflamed joints.

Posture requires special attention. In order to gain the patient's co-operation, the value of good, and the dangers of faulty posture, should be explained. The ideal position for the greater part of the day is lying on a firm mattress placed over fracture boards, with a single pillow under the head and a small one in the lumbar region, and a board at the feet projecting up vertically above the level of the toes. There should be no pillow under the knees, and the arms should rest on pillows with some degree of abduction of the shoulders, and the wrist supported in a few degrees of extension. At least once daily, the patient should turn into prone lying to ensure maintenance of the lumbar curve and extension of the hips. When the patient sits up in bed, it is necessary to see that there is a firm back rest with the pillows arranged vertically and not in the 'arm-chair' position. If the patient is allowed to get up for periods during the day, careful attention should be paid to her posture and she should be taught to correct her position in front of a mirror so that she may see, and learn to feel, when it is correct. The feet should be included in any standing or walking postural exercises. Rhythmic contractions of the main muscle groups are added and the exercises are gradually progressed. Breathing exercises are most important to aid the posture of the chest as well as to stimulate the circulation. General and local chest expansion should both be taught.

Training in relaxation is essential if full rest is to be obtained. Nearly all patients are tense, partly due to worry and partly to continuous pain. The first step is to explain what is meant by relaxation and its value, and this is followed by an attempt to find a position in which the patient is really comfortable and can relax. Usually the best method to follow is to teach the patient the difference between the 'feel' of contracted and relaxed muscles by starting on muscles and joints not as yet affected. Gradual progress can be made to painful joints. It will take patience and considerable time before any degree of relaxation can be obtained, but eventually it will be possible for the patient to relax completely.

Relief of symptoms and maintenance of the funtion of a joint. These are so closely related that the physical measures to fulfil these objects will be discussed together. They depend upon the condition of individual joints. For the purpose of selecting suitable treatment, joints may be classified

F

into four main groups, provided it is realised that there is no clear line of distinction between each group, and that a joint may be in one group at one time and in another later.

The acute joint. Joints in this state usually present with continuous pain and extreme tenderness, so that the patient can hardly bear to have the joint touched; muscle spasm resulting in complete absence of movement; swelling; heat and a tendency to hold the joint in the position of ease. The first principle of treatment for such a joint is rest and this is usually obtained by splintage. As the joint improves, attention should be paid to residual pain, stimulation of absorption of inflammatory exudate, prevention of muscle atrophy and deformity. Rhythmic muscle contractions should be taught and gentle assisted active movements carried out within the limit of real pain. Gradually as the inflammation subsides, the splint can be discarded until it is worn only at night

The active but non-acute joint. Probably the greater number of joints are found in this stage. The characteristics are pain, which is not continuous, but tends to be troublesome in the morning, at night and on movement; tenderness is still present, but it is not elicited so easily and the patient is able to tolerate light handling of the joint; the range of movement is greater but is not by any means full, and often muscle spasm will be precipitated when a certain point in the movement is reached; the muscles show considerable atrophy; swelling is marked and feels soft and spongy since it is usually rather the result of granulation tissue growth than of effusion; deformity is often present, though it is not yet a fixed deformity. More vigorous treatment is now necessary, but it must be carried out with care, avoiding anything which might stimulate the inflammatory process.

The main objects now are to prevent organisation of the granulation tissue, to build up the muscles, to protect the joint, and to prevent deformities becoming permanent. To carry out the first object, stimulation of the deep circulation is necessary and wax is probably the method of choice where possible. Carefully chosen active movements are essential to fulfil the second and third aims. Slings, proprioceptive facilitation, maximal resistance techniques and general treatment in the pool all have their place. The physiotherapist must select the most suitable treatment for each particular patient and be guided by her reactions as to how much she can do, gently pushing her on, but being wary of causing a flare-up of pain and inflammation. The patient should also be taught some simple exercises that she can do by herself. Particular attention is necessary to prevent deformities developing as the result of pain, muscle spasm and muscle weakness. Thus it is particularly important to exercise the lumbricales to prevent toe clawing, and if necessary, faradism may be used to start the retraining of these muscles. It must be remembered that muscles do not work alone: for example, an arthritic knee joint will not affect the quadriceps alone, but also probably the hamstrings, glutei, and feet which should all be watched and treated if necessary. Splints can again be a valuable aid.

The chronic joint, when the disease is still active. This joint is usually no longer painful at rest because the inflammatory process has, for the time being, at least, subsided. It may, however, be painful on movement as a result of fibrous tissue contracture and irregularity of joint surfaces. Tenderness on pressure and along the joint line is, for the same reason, no longer likely to be present, but there is often localised tenderness over tight tendon or ligamentous attachments. The joint is still swollen but the swelling is firmer since it is caused by fibrous thickenings. Movement is usually limited as a result of contractures and habit spasm of muscles; occasionally ankylosis may have occurred. Deformity and gross muscle atrophy are most commonly present.

The chief objects of treatment are very similar to the previous group, but as the inflammation is no longer present, they can be pressed rather further.

Localised tender areas, often causing considerable discomfort, can quite often be cleared by a few treatments using counter-irritant measures such as Renotin ionisation, strong localised doses of ultra-violet rays or deep frictions. The position of the joints can in many cases be improved, though not fully corrected, in the following way. The soft tissues are first warmed, softened and relaxed by the use of heat, inductothermy often proving the most successful. Stretching can then be attempted by means of deep massage, and active assisted exercises. Proprioceptive facilitation techniques are excellent, as very often a patient will have forgotten how to use muscles in the proper pattern or will be afraid to use a muscle maximally unless she is confident that the physiotherapist's hand will stop her jarring and hurting the joint. Weights should be used with great care for rheumatoid arthritis, especially if the patient has osteoporosis. The need for home exercises cannot be over emphasised.

It is important to remember that so long as the disease is active, it is possible by faulty treatment to re-start an inflammation in the joint. For this reason, forced movements are not permitted and any movement causing real pain is avoided.

The chronic joint when the disease has burnt itself out. The real point at issue in this stage is whether any improvement of the joint condition is possible. In some, useful improvement can be obtained as the patient's health is improving and she can tolerate more vigorous treatment following the lines of the previous group.

In others, it is a matter of training the patient to make the best use of what function, if any, remains, and she can often be helped to lead a happier, more independent life by the provision of suitable equipment.

When it is suggested to a patient that she should use splints, aids, sticks or crutches, she often objects that this will result in her joints becoming stiff and in an inability to do the things which she can still do. This, of course, is not true, provided the appliances are suitably used.

Aids may be considered as equipment which enables a patient to do things which she could not do before. After assessment it may be realised that for a considerable period the patient has not been able to wash the back of her neck or do her hair: twisted combs and long-handled brushes may make all the difference. The fingers may be so crippled that she cannot turn on taps or unscrew jars: gadgets are available to make these tasks possible. It is essential that the physiotherapist should find out what the patient cannot do and then try to see if there is any equipment that will help, and here co-operation with the occupational therapist is valuable.

Another problem is that of sticks and crutches. Patients do not usually like these because they feel that if they once start using them, they will not walk without their aid again. Often it is necessary to explain that sticks or crutches will help by sharing the weight between the arms and legs, so taking some of the strain from the affected leg joints. Sometimes the hands are unsuitable for sticks, and elbow (or gutter) crutches are most useful. Whatever is ordered, it is essential to see that they are the right length and being properly used.

It is also sometimes encouraging to explain to the patient that as she improves, she may no longer require the various aids and they can be handed back. It is a mistake to use them longer than is absolutely necessary.

Splints are used to rest, support or to prevent deformity in an arthritic joint, and can be made of plaster of Paris, polythene, leather, metal or a combination such as a leather T-strap with an iron to support the ankle.

The splints most usually made by the physiotherapist are plaster gutter splints and are kept in place either by crêpe bandages, which allow the limb to swell or reduce in size; or by webbing straps fastened with Velcro. The patient should be told that she will not stiffen up in the splint, but on the contrary, be able to relax into it, which will rest the joint and ease the pain.

Hands and wrists are usually splinted in the position of rest; that is, with the wrist slightly extended, the fingers gently flexed, and the thumb slightly flexed and opposed so that it rests under the index finger as though the hand were about to grasp a ball. The splint should be sufficiently raised along the outer border of the little finger to prevent ulnar deviation of the fingers.

Resting splints for the carpal tunnel syndrome are made in the neutral position and some physicians prefer them on the dorsum of the hand and forearm. Working splints of polythene, which support the wrists, leaving the thumb and fingers free, are a great help to patients. These should also be made with the wrist slightly extended to enable them to grasp things properly.

Splints for the knee are mainly used to correct or prevent flexion and a valgus deformity which sometimes develops in arthritics. Plaster cylinders are applied with the knee in as much extension as the patient can do actively, and these are either changed at fortnightly intervals or the plaster can be bi-valved and kept on with crêpe bandages. Rheumatoid knees are sometimes manipulated at fortnightly intervals and put in plaster cylinders to straighten them when other methods have failed. The patient must be encouraged to wear the splint all the time. As the knee improves, a gutter splint at night may be all that is necessary.

Polythene cages are used to support the knee during the day, and while walking, if the quadriceps are very weak and the joint painful.

Collars may also be required for patients who have suffered a subluxation of a cervical vertebra, the object being to support the head and neck and allow stabilisation to take place, thus attempting to avert increasing pressure on the cord or its blood supply.

They are also used to rest an acutely painful neck, as in cervical spondylosis. Collars, made by the physiotherapist, are of thick felt with polythene stiffeners or Sorbo rubber, while the instrument makers use polythene.

LENGTH OF COURSE OF PHYSIOTHERAPY

It is not possible to say exactly how long a patient should be treated as each case varies. In general it may be said that the object is to teach the patient how best to help herself so that she can carry on at home. One of the most important points is to teach her the relationship of rest and exercise. It is clearly stressed that when a joint is really painful at rest, it needs rest and the splints provided for this purpose should be worn and the joint saved as much as possible. As the pain subsides, exercise should be re-started, at first without weight. In selecting exercises during a course of treatment, stress is laid on those which can be done at home without apparatus. It is also wise to limit the number of exercises, as usually the patient cannot remember very many, and to give definite instruction as to how often the exercises should be done and for how long. The patient can be taught to use heat lamps and wax at home. As long as the patient needs a form of treatment which cannot be done safely at home and as long as her full co-operation and understanding have not been obtained, she needs to attend the department. Thus, one patient may require only a few weeks of treatment; another, months. Usually it is found that a course of about three months may be followed by a return to work but with assiduous practice of home exercises. Often the patient returns for another course during exacerbations.

THE ATTITUDE OF THE RELATIVES

In the early stages of the illness, the relatives are usually kind, helpful and considerate. Often, in fact, too much is done for the patient, and in an effort to make her comfortable, wrong treatment is given. Quite often, for example, the patient is nursed with a pillow under the knees producing a flexion deformity. Later the relative may get rather tired of a depressed, frustrated sufferer and sympathy and tact are not conspicuous, and here co-operation with the medical social worker is useful.

It is not usually the physiotherapist's place to deal with the relatives, but occasionally a word of advice is asked for and should be given. It is necessary, therefore, to have an understanding of the difficulties and of the way in which the relatives can help.

SURGERY

Surgery in rheumatoid arthritis is undertaken to relieve pain, to improve or restore function, or to correct deformity. Before deciding whether a patient is suitable for operation, the surgeon will consider the patient's temperament and in some cases her weight, as well as her general health, as it is obvious that some will make every effort to get on, while others do not co-operate to their fullest extent. The patient will have been told what the surgeon proposes to do, and if possible will have met someone who has already had the same operation and is happy with the result.

When patients are on steroids, special care is taken and the dose is increased temporarily (the steroid 'umbrella') as they cannot draw on their own adrenal supplies to help them withstand the stress of an operation.

Synovectomy. The removal of diseased synovium in the hand and wrist is preferably undertaken in the very early stages of rheumatoid arthritis, before any erosions of bone are seen radiologically, and therefore before severe damage has been done to joints, tendons and tendon sheaths.

In more advanced arthritis, the tendons in the hand (usually the long extensors of the fingers) may rupture due to either the invasion of the tendon sheaths by granulation tissue or to the roughening of the bone ends over which the tendons pass. The tendons can be sutured, repaired with a nylon gap suture, or be transplanted or grafted.

Physiotherapy is given to prevent adherence to underlying structures and to restore function. Wax, followed by massage, gentle frictions round the scar and active exercises should be given.

Synovectomy is also carried out on the knee when movement is good but pain and swelling are present.

Median nerve compression (carpal tunnel syndrome) by synovial hypertrophy is relieved by incision of the transverse carpal ligament, when splinting and injections of hydrocortisone have failed.

Arthrodesis, which has already been discussed in the surgical treatment of osteo-arthrosis, is also used successfully in rheumatoid arthritis, particularly in the hip, knee and wrist. It can also be carried out on the metacarpophalangeal joint of the thumb and interphalangeal joints of the fingers to render them more stable, and on the toes to straighten out clawing, though some surgeons prefer to remove them.

Arthroplasty and osteotomy are not as successful in rheumatoid arthritis as in osteo-arthrosis as the rheumatoid patient's muscles are rarely strong enough to control the joint and render it stable. These techniques are, therefore, more successful in non-weight-bearing joints such as the elbow.

STILL'S DISEASE

This is an acute systemic form of rheumatoid disease occurring in children. It is very similar to the adult type, but differs in that it is more severe. More joints are involved, the lymphoid tissue throughout the body is enlarged, and the constitutional reaction is much greater. The disease may begin insidiously in the joints, but more usually there is a high fever, a rash and a high sedimentation rate.

There may be an interval between the systemic and the arthritic involvement but usually the muscles are very tender and the joints acutely inflamed, making the child very unwilling to be handled. As a rule the young patient lies in bed, tense and frightened, a picture of misery. The heart, eyes and liver may also be involved. Often the joints of the neck are affected so that there is considerable danger of flexion deformity of the cervical spine.

Particular care should be taken of the posture in bed and the child should be encouraged to lie on the face every day for a brief period in order to avoid flexion contractures of the hip. If necessary joints such as the wrist should be splinted in a good, functional position as there is a danger of fibrous ankylosis.

The condition usually persists for several years and when it burns itself out, it leaves the child with much crippling and deformity. The treatment follows very closely that for the adult form of rheumatoid arthritis. As with adults, rest and analgesics are the first choice of treatment, and spontaneous remission may occur. It is not always maintained, however, and children are then given steroids as well as aspirin.

From the physiotherapist's point of view, treatment consists of splinting to prevent deformities, heat to relieve pain and active movements to maintain joint function. Hydrotherapy is the treatment *par excellence* as the patient can enjoy herself in the pool, while building up muscle power and increasing joint range.

FELTY'S SYNDROME

This is an arthritis of the rheumatoid type, having in addition enlargement of the spleen, decrease of white blood corpuscles and brown pigmentation of the skin, associated with weight loss and bouts of fever.

SJÖGREN'S SYNDROME

This is a polyarthritis of the rheumatoid type associated with dryness of the eyes and mouth. The upper respiratory and gastro-intestinal tracts are also affected so that patients are liable to infections of the respiratory tract and have difficulty in swallowing.

REITER'S SYNDROME

Reiter's syndrome is a disease of young men who develop a polyarthritis associated with non-specific urethritis, conjunctivitis and sometimes a skin rash. The disease may be acquired venereally, or may follow bacillary dysentery. The ankles, knees and feet are most commonly affected, demonstrating a subacute inflammatory arthritis. Occasionally the hips, sacro-iliac joints and spine are affected (when it resembles a spondylitis), as are also the upper limbs.

SYSTEMIC (DISSEMINATED) LUPUS ERYTHEMATOSUS

This is a generalised connective tissue disease which may affect any or all the systems of the body.

The cause is unknown, but it is thought to be due to a derangement of the body's immunological mechanism, since a number of serum factors have been identified which appear to be antibodies to the nucleo-protein of cells.

Systemic lupus erythematosus occurs mainly in young and middle-aged women and may follow discoid lupus or rheumatoid arthritis or appear apparently spontaneously. It mimics a large number of other conditions, the commonest symptoms being fever, malaise, arthralgia (which is often more painful than would appear from the changes apparent), weight loss, proteinurea, lymphadenopathy, enlargement of the liver and spleen, a butterfly rash on the face, psychiatric abnormalities, a high sedimentation rate, lupus erythematosus cells in the blood and a false-positive Wassermann and Kahn test. The course of the disease is variable and usually episodic, some cases being mild with long periods of remission, others severe, progressive and fatal within a few weeks or months.

SCLERODERMA

This is a chronic, systemic sclerosis affecting women more than men, usually between the ages of thirty and fifty.

The patient presents a picture of thickening and loss of elasticity of the skin and connective tissue in the hands, feet, arms, legs, face, neck and torso, with Raynaud's phenomenon in hands, and less commonly in the feet. The skin gradually contracts so that the face loses all expression, and the hands look and feel as though they had been fitted into a skin two sizes too small. There may be a vascular necrosis of the whole or part of the toes and fingers, with ulceration of the hands, feet or legs. The tips of the fingers become shortened, and the ends of the terminal phalanges become absorbed. The muscles become weak and atrophic, secondary to the fixed inelastic contraction of the surrounding structures. Thus flexed, fixed joints develop with, in the majority of cases, no intra-articular changes. Visceral changes usually follow the skin changes; the lungs, kidneys and heart, and the gastro-intestinal tract, become involved and the patient becomes more and more exhausted and undernourished. Remissions may occur, but slow relentless progression is more usual.

POLYARTERITIS NODOSA

(Synonym: periarteritis nodosa, polyarteritis necrotising angiitis)

This condition affects men between the ages of twenty and sixty-five more than women. Polyarteritis nodosa is a collagen disease in which the small and medium-sized arteries become involved in an inflammatory process ending in necrosis.

The lesions are most commonly situated at the bifurcation of the arteries, though veins may also be affected. All the coats of the vessel are involved, the nodules being formed by chronic peri-arterial inflammation and fibrosis, or by the formation of an aneurysm secondary to the fibrosis, which may lead to a fatal haemorrhage. In some cases no nodules are seen.

As with all other collagen diseases, the symptoms are variable and widespread, and may arise in any system or organ of the body. The onset may be gradual or sudden, the course fulminant or remittant; but the prognosis is generally poor though remissions have been known to occur.

The treatment for systemic lupus erythematosus, scleroderma and polyarteritis nodosa can be grouped together.

It is essentially palliative. The patient is advised to avoid over-fatigue and stress. Steroids and analgesics are given, and where necessary, antibiotics for local infections.

From the physiotherapist's point of view, treatment is mainly symptomatic and directed at relieving pain.

CHAPTER 4

Ankylosing Spondylitis

ANKYLOSING SPONDYLITIS IS a disease characterised by rigidity of the spinal column and thorax, often associated with considerable deformity. There has been much discussion as to whether it is simply a form of rheumatoid arthritis affecting the spine or whether it is a separate entity. In this country, it is usually considered to be a separate disease. This opinion is based on the fact that the sex incidence, joints affected and main changes are dissimilar; though its inflammatory nature, the general ill health, the anaemia and raised sedimentation rate are all symptoms present in rheumatoid arthritis. This condition, unlike rheumatoid arthritis, does not respond to gold therapy.

The condition affects men more than women, the usual age of onset being fifteen to forty. Cases occurring in later life are reported but it is probable that in these patients the condition has actually been present for some years before it was diagnosed.

The cause of the condition is unknown. The onset of symptoms is often related, by the patient, to some slight injury, such as a fall or a blow on the back, and he complains of pain. The proximal joints are affected first. Almost invariably it begins in the sacro-iliac joints and spreads up the spine (Plate VIII), eventually including the thoracic and cervical spines, sometimes producing a subluxation of the atlanto-axial joint, and immobilising the ribs. The condition may spread to the shoulders and downwards to the hips and occasionally to the knees. It but rarely affects the small distal joints although sometimes changes do occur similar to those seen in rheumatoid arthritis.

CHANGES

There is uncertainty as to the exact series of changes which are taking place, but in advanced cases the most definite change which can be seen in X-ray films is bony ankylosis. This is caused by calcification in the capsule and ligaments and in the edges of the articular cartilage and intervertebral discs. Eventually the articular surfaces are often joined by soft spongy bone and the ligaments become completely ossified, culminating in the 'bamboo' spine. The lateral ligaments, the supra- and interspinous ligaments, the anterior longitudinal ligament and ligamenta flava are particularly affected. The ligaments of the costo-vertebral and costo-transverse joints are also attacked. At the hip calcification begins in the acetabular labrum and spreads to the capsule.

MODE OF ONSET AND PROGRESS

The onset of the disease is often insidious. Sometimes there is a pre-spondylitic phase, developing between the ages of about fourteen and twenty, in which there is a complaint of stiffness and vague pains in the legs and trunk. Sometimes there is malaise and a slight pyrexia. Usually these symptoms disappear rapidly. If the patient is examined at this stage, the sacro-iliac joints will probably show a bilateral arthritis. Some years later there will be aching and stiffness in the lumbar region. Usually this increases gradually until the lumbar region may have become completely ankylosed. Sometimes remissions occur and these may last for years. It is not uncommon after a period of quiescence for the condition to recur in the thoracic or cervical regions. In some cases the disease progresses until the spine and chest and even the hips are completely rigid.

SIGNS AND SYMPTOMS

Pain is a fairly constant feature though it varies in the time of onset; some patients have almost complete rigidity of the lumbar spine before the onset of pain. Aching discomfort and pain are usually first felt in the lumbar region, since the condition almost invariably commences in the sacro-iliac and lumbar joints. Gradually with the spread of the arthritis, pain extends up the whole back. Many patients complain of pain round the chest and abdomen or pain extending into the limbs, which is worse on jarring, and sciatica is an occasional complaint. These pains are the result of irritation of the spinal nerves, or are referred from spinal segments into the area of distribution of these segments. If limb joints are involved, pain is also felt in relation to these joints. *Tenderness* can sometimes be elicited by gentle pressure over the spinous processes or adjacent muscles.

Limited movement is an early feature in whatever joints are involved, due to the inflammatory changes. In the limb joints the progress of the arthritis is extraordinarily rapid, and fibrous or bony ankylosis results in complete loss of movement. In the spine, rigidity of the affected area may be partly masked by movement in neighbouring regions, but if the patient is carefully watched, a flattening of the affected area on movement can be easily recognised. Joints between the ribs and vertebrae, early involved, quickly

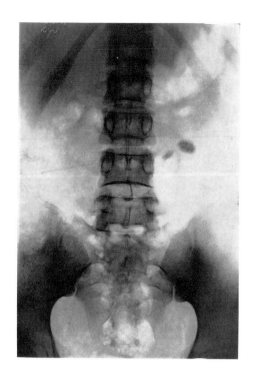

PLATE VIII (*see p. 73*)

ANKYLOSING SPONDYLITIS

(a) Early case. Showing bilateral sacro-iliac arthritis. Note sclerosis and loss of joint space in right joint. No evidence of changes in spine

(b) Advanced case. Note continuous outline of right side of vertebral column showing calcification of ligaments

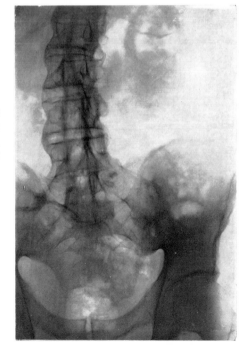

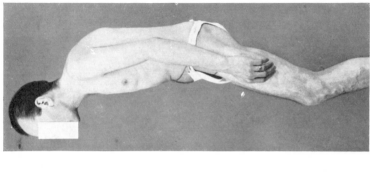
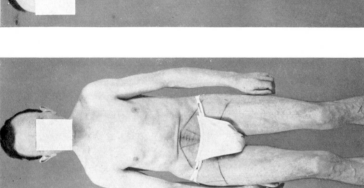
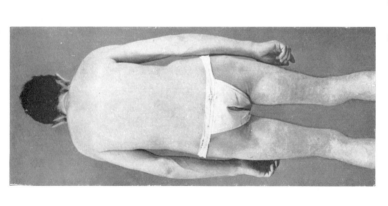

PLATE IX. ANKYLOSING SPONDYLITIS (*see p. 75*)

Showing deformity in advanced case. Note emaciation, flexion deformity, position of head, scoliosis, flat lumbar spine, diminished costal angle

stiffen and a much diminished thoracic mobility is soon apparent, progressing until respiration becomes entirely abdominal.

Deformity in ankylosing spondylitis varies very much from case to case and no adequate explanation of this can be given. It seems that whatever treatment is undertaken, some patients will eventually develop a severe flexion deformity of the spine and hips while others retain a remarkably good posture. All cases show loss of lumbar concavity (see Plate IX).

If one hip joint is affected, there is nearly always a scoliosis also. Practically every patient suffers from a flattening of the chest, diminution of the costal angle and decreased width of the intercostal spaces, these thoracic changes hampering the action of lungs and heart and causing laxity of the abdominal wall. If the cervical spine is involved, increase in the cervical concavity causes the head to be carried forward on the shoulder while the chin is thrust out. The dorsal curve is usually increased.

The general health is poor. Nearly all patients are under-weight and look and feel ill during the long active stage. The blood sedimentation rate is high and as long as it remains raised, the condition may be considered to be active. Owing to the impairment of the action of the lungs, chest complications are very likely and bronchitis is a common feature. Iritis is another fairly common complication of this disease.

EXAMINATION OF THE PATIENT

Before commencing physiotherapy, a thorough examination of the patient must be carried out. This may be conducted on the lines discussed for rheumatoid arthritis but the mobility of the thorax should be tested also and records of weight, chest expansion and vital capacity made. Where there is much deformity, a spinal tracing should be taken or the curve measured with a spondylometer. It is of value to see the X-ray photographs in order that the presence of bony ankylosis or calcification of ligaments may be noted.

TREATMENT

There is so far no cure for ankylosing spondylitis, but aspirin in some form, Butazolidin and deep X-ray are used to control the pain.

X-ray therapy. It is felt by many authorities that the relief from pain far outweighs the remote chance of leukaemia developing as a result of radiation. Relief usually occurs within a week or two of starting X-ray treatment, and physiotherapy in the form of general mobility exercises can be given concurrently, always within the limit of pain.

Contra-indications after X-ray therapy. Heat should not be given for at least six months after radiation or while pigmentation persists, as the condition of the skin is not suitable. Most authorities prefer patients not to start pool exercises for about two months after treatment by X-ray therapy, because of the action of water on the skin.

Physiotherapy should commence as soon as possible since once calcification has occurred no further movement in that region can be obtained. These patients are encouraged to lead as normal a life as possible, and treatment is given in a class so that suitable easy games can be introduced into the scheme of exercises. Pool therapy is particularly valuable as the warmth of the water assists the patient to relax. Particular care should be given to the hip joints. A rigid spine is not too great a handicap, providing the posture is reasonably good, but ankylosed hips are severely disabling. Breathing exercises must always be given, though no improvement in mobility may be obtained, so that chest diseases are less likely to arise.

Home exercises. Very careful instruction and explanation of their purpose and value must be given, particularly stressing the importance of relaxation and breathing exercises. The patient should be told to sleep on his back on a firm mattress, using only one pillow, and if possible, to spend half an hour at midday lying flat.

PROGNOSIS

While very occasionally ankylosing spondylitis may follow a rapidly progressive course and result in total incapacity in two or three years, in the great majority of cases the prognosis for life appears to be little affected and function is much better than might be expected. Thus pain tends usually to diminish, and the constitutional disturbance to abate as the spine becomes increasingly rigid. The severity of the hip involvement and the patient's morale are major factors in determining his ultimate functional capacity. Atlanto-axial subluxation occurs in some advanced spondylitics producing neurological signs.

SURGERY

The results of arthroplasty for ankylosis of the hip have not been as successful as in osteo-arthrosis. Wedge osteotomy can be done to correct a severe flexion deformity of the spine.

CHAPTER 5

Non-articular Rheumatism

FIBROSITIS AS A DIAGNOSIS is less used now that knowledge of psychogenic rheumatism, referred pain and specific shoulder syndromes increases. Following unaccustomed exercise pain spots may develop in the deltoid and persist for months. Diffuse tenderness in many muscle groups without any obvious cause, may be due to referred pain (c.f. cervical spondylosis), or poor posture. Many patients, however, complain of pain brought on by damp, cold and draughts, which may be due to muscle spasm producing temporary ischaemia. Tension, the result of stress and anxiety, produces pain particularly in the shoulder girdle, and in this case the value of relaxation should be explained to the patient, and she should be taught how to practise at home, and given some simple exercises to strengthen the affected muscles. Heat and massage make the patient more comfortable temporarily, but do not touch the cause of the condition.

EXAMINATION OF THE PATIENT

It is absolutely essential to try to find the exact site of the lesion so that treatment can be directed to this and not to the site of referred pain.

It is important to take a careful history, particularly noting where the pain was first felt, since this is usually a true guide to the site of the lesion. Observation is important in order to note the general appearance and posture. The presence of spasm, of swelling and changes of colour should all be noted. The way the patient holds the affected part is a useful sign. Changes in muscle tone, swelling or atrophy can be particularly well detected by the sense of touch and generalised tenderness can also be appreciated at the same time. Palpation for trigger points should not be carried out until the movements have been tested.

Test of movement is the most important part of the examination. Where pain is referred, each joint within the area supplied by the segment of the spinal cord should be tested. If pain is felt in the arm, movement of fingers, wrist, forearm, elbow, neck, shoulder girdle and shoulder should all be examined. Each movement which can normally be carried out in the joint should be tested passively and actively. The patient should then be asked to try to perform the movement against such resistance that it will ensure that no movement actually occurs in the joint. In this case no structure is stretched but certain muscles contract strongly. While the movements are being tested note should be made of pain, limitation by muscle spasm, or unusual sounds such as snapping, clicking or crepitus.

The actual findings in the examination will enable the lesion to be isolated to a certain structure. First, if there is pain on passive and active movement in the same direction, an inert structure such as the capsule is at fault. Secondly, if pain occurs on active movement in one direction and passive in the reverse, a muscle or tendon is probably concerned, and should pain arise when such resistance is given so that no movement occurs, the lesion is definitely in a contractile structure. The significance of these findings was first pointed out by Cyriax, and there are many other points which arise and which are of value in estimating the exact location of the lesion. For a full account of these reference should be made to his book, *Rheumatism and Soft Tissues Injuries*.

When a lesion has been tracked to a definite structure careful palpation should be made to find a tender spot. If pressure on such a spot reproduces the patient's pain, then it is probably the real lesion.

It will be remembered that the articular surfaces of the shoulder joint are surrounded by a loose capsule with which are blended the tendons of supraspinatus, infraspinatus, teres minor and subscapularis. These four tendons form a cuff round the joint and are often spoken of as the rotator cuff (Fig. 1). Covering the greater tuberosity and blending with the rotator cuff is the subacromial bursa separating these structures from the deltoid muscle. In addition the bursa extends up beneath the acromion, protecting the supraspinatus tendon from constant friction. The floor of the bursa is adherent to the supraspinatus, coraco-humeral ligament and the capsule, while the roof is adherent to the under surface of the coraco-acromial arch; thus as the humerus moves in the glenoid cavity, the upper part of the joint moves in relation to the arch, and ease and freedom of movement are guaranteed.

SUBACROMIAL BURSITIS

Subacromial bursitis may be the result of trauma or may occur in rheumatoid arthritis, in which condition the bursae are particularly liable to be inflamed; or it may develop insidiously. When the bursa is affected it swells and gets nipped between the supraspinatus tendon and the acromion process when the arm is raised sideways, producing a typical painful arc, between about 60° and 100°. The condition usually yields to conservative

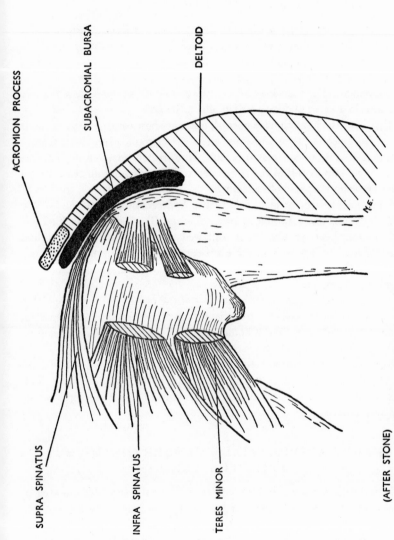

ACROMION PROCESS

SUBACROMIAL BURSA

DELTOID

SUPRA SPINATUS

INFRA SPINATUS

TERES MINOR

(AFTER STONE)

Fig. 1. Posterior aspect of the right shoulder joint.

G

treatment following the lines for frozen shoulder, but occasionally excision of the bursa or the acromion may be necessary.

FROZEN SHOULDER

This is a severe periarthritis (capsulitis) usually affecting patients over forty, which can follow trauma, or cardiovascular, pulmonary or metabolic disease, or appear spontaneously. It is characterised by pain which becomes progressively more acute, tenderness, muscle spasm and gross restriction of movement. The pain may be so acute as to compel the patient to carry her arm in a sling, and may radiate down the arm.

On X-ray the joint appears normal, but may show osteoporosis. Sections taken from postmortems show necrotic areas surrounded by inflammatory reaction, that is, a degenerated capsule. If untreated the joint may become completely stiff owing to the fibrinous exudate gumming up the synovial membrane and capsule of the joint.

The usual treatment is an injection of hydrocortisone into the joint to allay inflammation, followed by physiotherapy. This consists of either ice, ultrasonics, heat or shortwave followed by stabilisations, pendulum movements, pulleys and active exercises, all within the painfree range. Hydrotherapy is very useful for shoulders that are unresponsive to other forms of treatment.

In the chronic stage gentle stretching of the capsule, though painful at the time, produces relief after treatment. It must be impressed on the patient that she must do exercises at home in spite of the pain. The condition can last from four months to two years.

Bicipital tendinitis is a frequent complication of frozen shoulders, the most painful spot being where the tendon lies in the bicipital groove. This can be greatly helped by injections of hydrocortisone, or if of long standing, by deep frictions.

RUPTURE AND PARTIAL RUPTURE OF THE SUPRA-SPINATUS TENDON

The immediate cause may be a sudden strain of the shoulder followed by pain and weakness. In older patients, the tendon may rupture slowly following unaccustomed movements, possibly because of pre-existing degenerative changes. The aim of treatment is to control pain and restore normal movement and therefore follows the pattern for frozen shoulders.

PART III

Diseases of the Respiratory System

REVISED BY

E. A. BEAZLEY, M.C.S.P., Dip.T.P.

CHAPTER 1

Introduction. Signs and Symptoms.
Examination of the Patient.
Principles of Treatment

I T IS NOT WITHIN THE SCOPE of a book of this nature to describe in detail the structure and function of the respiratory apparatus, but certain points do deserve special consideration if the physiotherapist is to work intelligently in the chest unit.

THE PLEURAL SAC. The lungs are each covered by a completely closed pleural sac, one layer of which lines the chest wall and floor, the other covering the lung. The layers are normally in contact, but move smoothly over one another owing to the small amount of serous fluid secreted by the epithelial cells of the membrane. However, a potential cavity does exist. Pressure within each pleural cavity is less than that of atmosphere. It varies below this point, rhythmically with respiration, dropping during inspiration and rising with expiration.

THE LUNGS are composed of a great number of lobules bound together by highly elastic connective tissue. Each lobule is a minature lung since it consists of a terminal bronchiole, ending in vestibule, atria, infundibulae and alveolar sacs, blood and lymph vessels and nerves. The lobules are joined together to form lobes.

DIVISION OF LUNGS INTO LOBES. Each lung is divided into two main lobes by an oblique fissure which passes posteriorly from the level of the third dorsal vertebra just above the hilum, laterally and downwards to the level of the fourth and fifth ribs in the mid-axillary line; then it continues anteriorly and downwards to end at the level of the sixth costal cartilage.

The upper lobe lying above this fissure includes the apex, anterior border, most of the medial surface and part of the costal surface. The lower lobe consists of the base, nearly all the posterior border and the rest of the costal surface. (See Fig. 2(A) and (B)).

The right lung has an additional transverse fissure, dividing the upper lobe into an upper and a lower, or middle lobe.

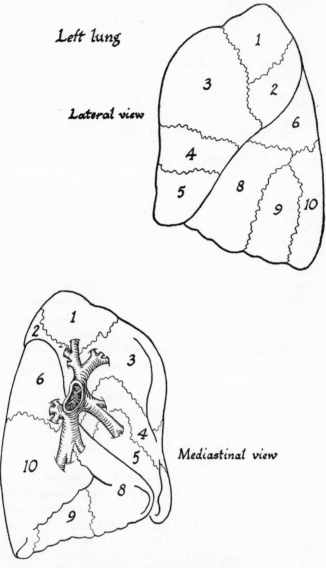

Fig. 2. A. Diagrammatic representation of the left broncho-
pulmonary segments.
(The numbers refer to the segments named in Fig. 2C)

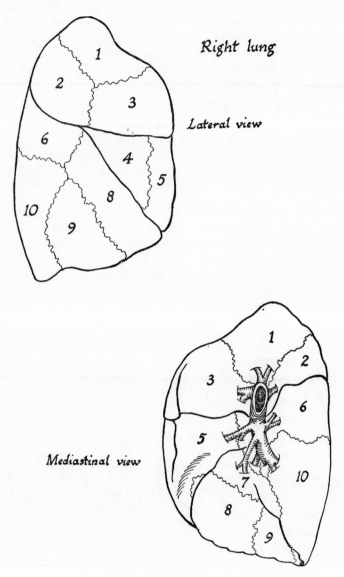

Right lung

Lateral view

Mediastinal view

Fig. 2. B. Diagrammatic representation of the right broncho-
pulmonary segments.
(The numbers refer to the segments named in Fig. 2c)

Every lobe consists of a number of segments, each having its own bronchus. Every segment is distinct from its fellow and occasionally this may be apparent on the surface of the lung by means of slight visible indentations. A knowledge of these segments is essential in both medical and surgical cases if these are to be treated effectively. The right lung is divided as follows (see Fig. 2C. I and II):

Upper lobe	Middle lobe	Lower lobe
Apical	Medial	Apical
Anterior	Lateral	Anterior basal
Posterior		Cardiac (medial basal)
		Lateral basal
		Posterior basal

The upper lobe bronchus divides into three. An apical bronchus passes up to supply the apical segment; a posterior bronchus passes backwards, laterally and slightly upwards to supply the posterior segment; and an anterior bronchus passes antero-laterally to the anterior segment.

The middle lobe bronchus passes forwards, laterally, and downwards, and divides into two to supply the medial and lateral segments of the middle lobe. The right lower lobe bronchus divides into five, the first of

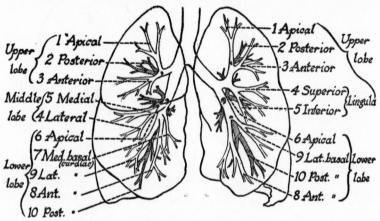

Fig. 2. c. (I) Diagram showing anterior view.

which passes exactly opposite the origin of the middle lobe, directly backwards into the apical segment of the right lower lobe. The others supply the four remaining segments of the lower lobe, that is the cardiac segment, anterior basal, lateral basal and posterior basal segments.

The left lung is very similar except that it has no middle lobe, this being represented by the lingula, neither is there a cardiac lobe. A further point of difference is that the apical bronchus of its upper lobe is more vertical, and its main upper lobe bronchus is more horizontal.

The left upper lobe bronchus gives off four main bronchi to five segments. The apical, anterior and posterior bronchi to the apical, anterior and posterior segments. The fourth is the lingular bronchus which divides into a superior and inferior branch to supply segments of the same name in the lingular area of the upper lobe. The lower lobe bronchus is similar to that of the right lower lobe except that it has four divisions instead of five since there is no cardiac segment on the left.

The left lung has nine segments, which are:

Upper lobe	*Lower lobe*
Apical	Apical
Anterior	Anterior basal
Posterior	Lateral basal
⟋Superior	
Lingula	Posterior basal
⟍Inferior	

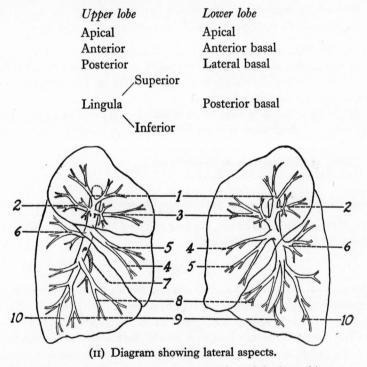

(ii) Diagram showing lateral aspects.

Fig. 2. C. Diagrammatic representation of the bronchi.

BRONCHI. In structure the bronchi consist of an outer coat of fibrous tissue and cartilage, a middle coat of smooth muscular tissue and an inner mucous coat which has a lining of ciliated columnar epithelium on a basement membrane. This inner coat contains a considerable quantity of elastic fibres and lymphoid tissue. As the tubes narrow and become smaller their structure gradually changes: no cartilage is found in the walls of bronchioles of less than one millimetre in diameter, and in these the muscular component is more evident. The ring of muscle forms sphincter-like structures at the end of the alveolar ducts. The lining of the alveoli is probably incomplete, and capillaries may push their way between the cells, consequently the blood is separated from the alveolar air by a membrane only one cell thick.

MECHANISM OF RESPIRATION

The thorax increases its dimensions in three directions:

Antero-posteriorly. The sternum is thrust forward by the upper ribs.
Laterally. Principally by the bucket handle action of the lower ribs.
Downwards. By the contraction of the diaphragm.

The lungs move with the ribs, and as the dimensions of the thorax are increased air is sucked into the main bronchi and so via their branches into the lungs. The muscles chiefly responsible for the act of quiet inspiration are the diaphragm and intercostals.

Respiration is said to have taken place when the interchange of gases has occurred. Expiration is normally a passive mechanism. The muscles relax and the chest wall returns to the resting position, simultaneously with the recoil of the elastic tissue of the lungs.

The respiratory rate is regulated by impulses from the respiratory centre which is subject to nervous and chemical factors.

The elastic tissue plays a very important part in normal quiet expiration; should the elastic recoil be lost, the lung will tend to remain expanded, and expiration becomes a positive act.

SECRETIONS

The cells of the mucous membrane lining the air passages from nose to respiratory bronchioles secrete small quantities of mucus, which moisten the tubes and help to trap small particles in the inspired air. There is a marked increase in mucus formation should this membrane be irritated in any way, when it may form a thick viscid layer over the surface, or may collect in the smaller tubes and act as a mucous plug preventing entry of air.

Dangers of excessive secretions

Should the excess mucus be allowed to remain certain complications may arise.

Atelectasis or collapse of the area of lung where air cannot enter because of the block, the air behind the block being gradually absorbed.

Infection. Bacteria may invade the stagnant mucus to form pus, thus causing a chronic inflammatory condition with consequent weakening of the tubal walls and eventual fibrosis.

Removal of excessive secretions

Normally these and foreign substances can be eliminated by coughing. The patient takes a deep breath and by closing the larynx, vigorously contracting the abdominal muscles to raise intra-pulmonary pressure, then relaxes the glottis to allow a sudden outflow of air to occur, carrying with it the offending substance.

This method would prove ineffective should all the air be absorbed behind a mucous plug, or should it be too deeply placed in the small tubes or alveoli so that no current of air can be behind it.

Provided the secretion is in that part of the tube proximal to the respiratory bronchiole, its movement upward is aided by the action of the cilia which will waft the substance into a region where coughing will be effective. Coughing may be suppressed if the cough reflex is inhibited as a result of an anaesthetic, or because the patient voluntarily inhibits coughing through fear of pain; the action of the cilia may cease because cold, or an anaesthetic decreases their activity, or as a result of a chronic inflammatory process where degeneration of the mucous membrane has occurred with loss of the ciliated epithelium. It is also possible that pus, mucus or inflammatory exudate is so viscid that it adheres to the walls of the tubes, or may have collected in cavities: in these cases the cough reflex becomes fatigued, and no nervous impulses are produced.

Certain steps must be taken to aid the expulsion of these secretions. Breathing exercises, percussion of the chest and agility exercises will help to loosen mucus, whilst gravity may be used to drain cavities. Sometimes suction drainage may be used.

POSTURAL DRAINAGE

This is the positioning of a patient so that the affected bronchus is in the most vertical position.

Upper lobe

Apical segment—upright

Anterior segment—lying flat on the back

Posterior segment—right lung: lying on opposite side turned about 45° towards the face

Left lung: sitting leaning forward with a 45° turn to the opposite side.

Middle lobe and lingular process

Middle lobe and lingular segments—lying on back but slightly turned to the opposite side, hips raised about 10 inches.

Lower lobe

Apical segment—patient lying flat on face

Anterior basal segment—patient lying on back, hips raised about 12 inches

Lateral basal segment—patient lying on opposite side, hips raised about 12 inches.

Posterior basal segment—patient lying on face, hips raised about 14 inches (*See* Figs. 3A, B, C, D, E, F, and G).

'Tipping' is done by raising the foot of the bed or plinth by means of a bed elevator, bed blocks, or a chair. Alternatively, or in addition, pillows may be used beneath the hips. In cases where the deepest 'tip' is required a Nelson bed may be used, or the patient may lean over the side of the bed with the hands on a stool, or the floor. This position is not very comfortable and should only be used if no other method is possible. In choosing the method and height of 'tip' attention must always be paid to the age and condition of the patient. Obviously a bronchiectatic child can stand a deeper and longer 'tip' than an elderly patient who has recently had a lobectomy.

BREATHING EXERCISES, PERCUSSION AND AGILITY

In some cases postural drainage alone is insufficient to move thick secretions. Purulent material, or viscid mucus, may sometimes be loosened and dislodged by doing agility exercises before 'tipping'. Any exercises which produce considerable movement in the trunk are useful, such as quick trunk forward and downward bending; trunk side flexion localising the movement to the thoracic spine as much as possible; brisk double arm circling; running and jumping. Obviously the age and condition of the patient have to be considered before agility work can be used.

Material can often be loosened by percussion on the chest wall. The patient is placed in the drainage position and vigorous shaking and clapping are given over the affected area of the lung; the strength of the percussion movements being modified according to the condition.

Deep breathing exercises will, by the movement of the lung tissue, help to dislodge accumulated material; particular emphasis being given to expiration. These exercises can be combined with percussion, and be carried out in the same position.

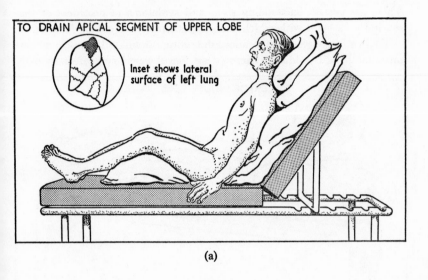

(a)

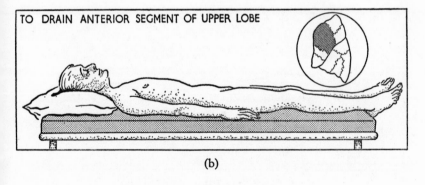

(b)

Fig. 3. Positions for postural drainage.

SIGNS AND SYMPTOMS OF RESPIRATORY DISORDERS

There are certain outstanding signs and symptoms of disorders of the respiratory system with which the physiotherapist should be familiar.

These are: cough, expectoration, dyspnoea, diminished thoracic movement and pain. In addition, haemoptysis, loss of weight and deformity may

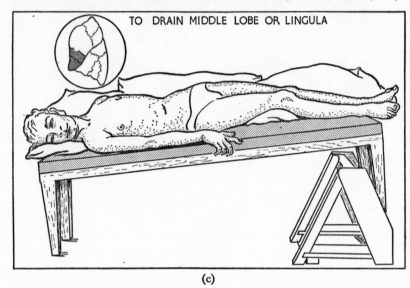

TO DRAIN MIDDLE LOBE OR LINGULA

(c)

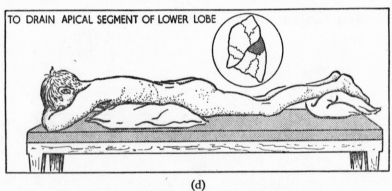

TO DRAIN APICAL SEGMENT OF LOWER LOBE

(d)

Fig. 3. Positions for postural drainage.

also be present. These symptoms do not necessarily indicate a respiratory lesion, in fact they may well be evidence of other diseases particularly cardiac, but they are likely to be present if disease occurs in the respiratory apparatus.

Cough. This may be a habit, or it may be the result of a reflex irritation. Thus, for example, disorders of the stomach may result in irritation of the afferent fibres of the vagus nerve and so cause a 'stomach' cough. Usually, however, a cough is due to irritation of the nerve endings in the mucous lining of the trachea and bronchi, either by mechanical irritants such as dust, smoke, a foreign body or a growth, or as a result of the action of bacteria causing an inflammatory reaction and increased secretion. In

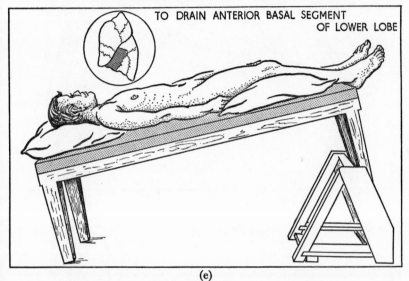

(e)

Fig. 3. Positions for postural drainage.

both cases the cough may be dry, or it may be accompanied by expectoration. The cough may show other characteristic features: it may be worse on change of posture, or at certain times of the day or night.

Expectoration. The sputum varies considerably both in quantity and appearance. It may be practically negligible, or may be in large quantities as often happens in lung abscess or bronchiectasis. If it appears clear in colour but viscid, it is mucoid sputum characteristic of irritation of the mucous membrane of larynx, trachea or main bronchi by such factors as smoke or dust. A scanty but stringy type of sputum usually occurs at the beginning of an acute infection, due to a fibrinous exudate. Purulent sputum will appear in severe infections, and is yellow or greenish in colour. If it is pink or reddish, this will be due to the presence of blood, which may be fresh or altered according to the length of time between haemorrhage and expectoration. It is not necessarily a serious sign to find evidence of blood in the sputum.

It is important to notice the amount and type of sputum and, if the patient is being treated by postural drainage, the amount expectorated during treatment should be carefully measured by the physiotherapist.

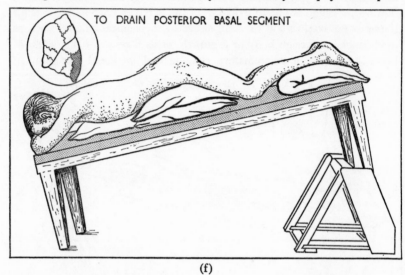

TO DRAIN POSTERIOR BASAL SEGMENT

(f)

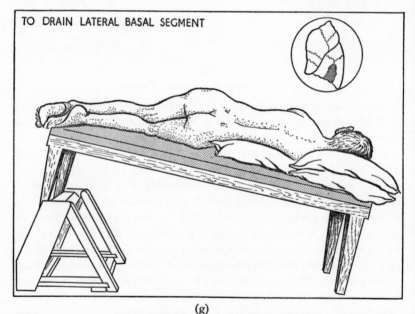

TO DRAIN LATERAL BASAL SEGMENT

(g)

Fig. 3. Positions for postural drainage.

Care must be taken not to confuse sputum with saliva, or with secretions from the naso-pharynx.

Dyspnoea. Coope defines dyspnoea as the 'word used to cover difficult, painful or disordered breathing'. Another term not quite so accurate, but in common use, is shortness of breath. It is not necessarily a sign of disease of the respiratory system. It may be, for example, a sign of cardiac or renal disease and it is also normally present in severe exercise. There are, however, many factors in respiratory disease which may be the cause of shortness of breath, these will include: loss of thoracic mobility, fibrosis or loss of elasticity of the lung tissue, narrowing of the bronchial tubes (these entailing greater effort on the part of the respiratory muscles to move the chest wall or lung, or to widen and lengthen the tubes), thickening of the alveolar lining where there is greater difficulty in absorbing oxygen, and finally low vital capacity where there is little interchange of gases. In both the last two cases the chemical factors influencing respiratory rate will be changed. Direct disturbance of the respiratory centre may also lead to dyspnoea.

Dyspnoea may be inspiratory, when it is due to obstruction to air entry, or expiratory, where there is bronchial spasm, or extensive loss of elasticity.

If dyspnoea is present with the patient lying, but relieved by sitting up, the term orthopnoea is used.

Pain in the thoracic region is again not necessarily proof of respiratory disease. The lung itself has no pain nerve endings and is therefore insensitive to pain. Either the pleura, ribs and thoracic muscles, the heart or the intercostal nerves may be affected if the patient complains of pain. If the pleura is inflamed the pain is of the sharp lancinating type, worse on each inspiration, so that the thoracic movement is restricted in that area. Pain, the result of muscular or bony lesion, may be very severe but all movements, not only respiratory, will increase it, and there will be localised tenderness and evidence of muscle spasm. Pain, due to involvement of the intercostal nerves will radiate along the course of the nerve. If pain is cardiac in origin, it will usually be felt behind the sternum, and may radiate up the left side of the neck and into the axilla, and the medial side of one or both arms.

Limited respiratory movements. Limitation in chest movements may be the result of a loss of elasticity of the lung tissue, resulting in fixation of the thorax in a position of inspiration. Again it may be the result of collapse, or fibrosis of one or more lobes resulting in diminished movement on one side of the chest; pleural adhesions may have the same effect. Shallow breathing results in little movement at the sides, posterior aspect and lower part of the chest wall.

H

It is important to realise that limited respiratory movements may be the result of other factors, such as ankylosing spondylitis, kyphosis, or scoliosis.

Haemoptysis. This term means the spitting of blood from the larynx, trachea, bronchi or lungs. If expectorated at once, it is unchanged and is generally bright red and frothy in appearance; such a haemoptysis is usually the result of a sudden rupture of a fairly large vessel in a tuberculous patch, or a bronchiectatic cavity. Blood coughed up may amount to several ounces. The sputum is usually streaked with blood for several successive days.

It is not uncommon to see minute quantities of blood in the sputum in acute inflammatory conditions of the lung, due to excessively dilated or ruptured capillaries.

Sometimes the blood is not coughed up at once, but is mixed with mucus or pus. It is then changed in colour, and may have a brownish red appearance, or may colour the sputum faintly pink.

Loss of weight. This is a feature of many diseases and does not necessarily occur in all respiratory disorders. It is, however, a feature of infective or malignant chest conditions and weight should therefore be carefully watched. Active tuberculosis, bronchiectasis and carcinoma are the three conditions in which weight is most likely to be lost.

Deformities. Although deformity is not in any way a diagnostic sign of respiratory disorders, many chest diseases are complicated by alteration in the shape of the thorax, by curvature of the spine and by inequality in the shoulder girdle. Difficulty in expiration, over use of the accessory muscles of respiration, imbalance of the muscles on either side of the chest and spine, painful conditions affecting one side of the chest, general poor muscle tone resulting from imperfect oxygenation of the blood, all these will lead to thoracic and spinal deformity. Expiratory dyspnoea leads to the chest being held in the position of forced inspiration. In time the muscles and ligaments will adapt themselves to this new position, and the chest will take on a barrel-shaped appearance in which the shoulders are high, the antero-posterior diameter of the thorax is as wide as the lateral, the costal angle is wide and the ribs are more horizontally placed.

Accessory muscles of respiration lift the upper ribs, and the neck appears unduly short and the shoulders high. These muscles are constantly in action if respiratory dyspnoea is present, and gradually they become shorter.

Muscle imbalance is a natural result of lack of movement of one side of the chest, or of chest surgery. Following a thoracoplasty, for example, extensive division of muscles is necessary, and one obvious deformity is the lateral shift of the trunk towards the sound side.

Unilateral painful respiratory conditions lead to deformities, because the patient tends to limit chest movement on the painful side and to lean to this side. In a pleurisy, therefore, a scoliosis is liable to develop its convexity towards the unaffected side.

In all respiratory conditions there is likely to be a decrease in gaseous interchange, and oxygenation of the blood may be incomplete. The metabolism of all the muscles of the body will, therefore, be impaired and their tone and strength is likely to be decreased. General posture is, as a result, defective and a general 'slump' develops to which any special fault arising from the particular chest condition may be added. A child suffering from bronchiectasis, for example, will in all probability show poor general posture, and in addition may show a thoracic scoliosis, particularly if the bronchiectatic condition is unilateral. The usual position is one in which the head is carried forward. This means that the muscles attaching to the clavicle and first rib (the scaleni and sterno-mastoid) are relaxed and the chest sinks forward, the costal angle is reduced, and the ribs are more vertical with narrowed intercostal spaces. Poor tone of the rhomboids allows the scapulae to glide forward, and the chest is then narrowed in its lateral diameters. All these thoracic deformities, though at first postural, become fixed as soft tissues adapt themselves to the new position. Respiration is, therefore, grossly affected.

EXAMINATION OF THE PATIENT PRIOR TO TREATMENT BY PHYSICAL MEASURES

A routine examination should be carried out in order to elicit certain essential facts. It is necessary before planning treatment to be aware of the state of general health, the extent of thoracic expansion and whether this is equal on both sides, and in some cases such as asthma and emphysema the vital capacity should be known. A knowledge of the range of movement obtainable in the joints of the thorax, spine and shoulder girdle is valuable, while details of any thoracic deformity should be known. It is essential to know if there is any cough, and if so whether it is productive, and the quantity and nature of the sputum.

Case notes and X-rays should be studied before proceeding to examination.

Interrogation. The patient is encouraged to recount the history of his illness and symptoms. This, together with his answers to questions, should elicit any important facts as regards the family history, his occupation, habits, home conditions, possible contact with infection, the presence of cough, sputum, pain and alterations in weight.

Observation. During the interrogation, certain points such as general appearance, colour, posture and health will have already been noted. A more detailed inspection is now carried out. The *shape of the chest* may first be considered. Normally the chest is wider from side to side than from back to front, and the diverging costal margins almost form a right angle with one another. Various changes may occur, the antero-posterior diameter may be increased, so that it equals the lateral and the chest assumes a barrel-shaped appearance. Alternatively, the antero-posterior diameter may be decreased, and the anterior aspect of the chest becomes flat instead of slightly convex. Hence the costal angle will be decreased, and the intercostal spaces diminished. Occasionally thoracic asymmetry may be noticed, i.e. either a flattening or a 'bulging' in one area. A localised flattening nearly always indicates some underlying lung disease, though it can be the result of muscle atrophy in a lower motor neurone lesion.

Abnormalities may also be present which are not the result of respiratory disease but which predisposes towards infection. Such may be the pigeon breast in which the sternum is thrust forward, and the sides of the chest flattened, a feature common in a case of rickets. A groove extending downwards from the sternum to axillary line, known as Harrison's sulcus, may be produced by the pull of the diaphragm on softened bone in the same condition.

Respiratory movements. These should be carefully watched. Note should be made of the type of breathing, apical or diaphragmatic, the depth and rate and whether or not the accessory muscles of respiration are being used. A careful check should be made to see if any particular area of the chest is moving less freely than the rest. Any sign of cyanosis or dyspnoea will be easily detected during this examination.

It is well also to examine the fingers since in chronic infective conditions 'clubbing' is often present.

Palpation. The physiotherapist should place her warm hands lightly on the chest, so checking any variations in thoracic movement on each side of the chest. Often slight differences in the amount of expansion can be better detected through palpation than observation. Any tenderness originating from lesions of bone or muscle will be noticed then also.

The range of movement of thoracic, vertebral and shoulder girdle joints should be tested next. If these joints have not been exercised to their full extent, owing to deformity or to diseases of the respiratory system, they will become permanently limited in range, so further reducing the possibility of good chest expansion and correct posture.

Measurements. The chest expansion should be measured. It is usual to take three measurements, *apical expansion* at the level of the angle of Louis, *lateral costal* at the level of the tip of the sternum and *diaphragmatic* at the level of the tip of the tenth rib. These measurements must be carefully recorded. The patient should be weighed and, if a spirometer is available, the vital capacity taken.

PRINCIPLES OF TREATMENT BY PHYSIOTHERAPY

Broadly speaking the chest diseases may be divided into acute conditions such as acute bronchitis, pleurisy and pneumonia, in which, at least during the acute phase, no physiotherapy is indicated, and chronic diseases such as chronic bronchitis, bronchiectasis, emphysema and asthma, where treatment by physical means can play an important part. A third group of cases are those which are going to have, or have had some surgical treatment. As these are surgical cases they will not be dealt with here.

THE CHRONIC CHEST CONDITIONS

All chronic chest conditions show certain characteristic features, particularly tenseness of neck and thoracic muscles, limited chest expansion, and reduced vital capacity; faulty breathing, defective posture, poor general health and in many cases cough with or without expectoration. The principles of treatment will, therefore, be similar but modified in their fulfilment according to the special features of each separate condition.

Relaxation

In most chest cases general and local tenseness is present. Difficult breathing engenders fear, and fear results in a condition of hypertonicity. This sets up a vicious circle because, as has already been seen, hypertonicity leads to an increased respiratory rate. Many patients with respiratory disorders are afraid, either that they may be suffering from conditions such as lung cancer, or tuberculosis, or that they may be unable to continue their work. An important step in treatment is, therefore, to find out what the patient is worrying about, and if possible to relieve him of this worry. This is, of course, done by the physician, but the patient often talks to the physiotherapist more freely, and any information in relation to such worries should be reported to the physician. The physiotherapist can also help by giving the patient very careful training in the art of relaxation. Both general and local relaxation require training because, in addition to general tenseness, if either inspiration or expiration requires special effort the accessory muscles of respiration are liable to be brought into action, and all muscles round the shoulder girdle show increased tone in order to give these muscles a firmer origin; much unnecessary tone is therefore present. Full relaxation of the neck and shoulder girdle muscles cannot, of course, be obtained until the breathing has improved, but much can be done to relieve unnecessary tenseness. In some cases the practice of relaxed head and shoulder movements will be of assistance.

Increase of chest expansion

This is a very important principle, since chest expansion is usually limited, either as a result of loss of elasticity of one or both lungs, or due to spasm of the bronchiole muscle, or through the presence of adhesions. Chest expansion can nearly always be increased by the use of breathing exercises. In the majority of chronic lung conditions better expansion will be gained by training the patient first in expiration. Where elasticity is lost, fuller expiration may be obtained by showing the patient how to give pressure on the chest by the use of a broad webbing belt, how to assist air exit from the lungs by relaxation of the chest and by movements of the trunk.

The second step, in gaining better expansion, is to teach the patient to use more fully those areas of the lung which are not being used to the best capacity. In most cases breathing is taking place at the upper part of the chest, so that by use of manual pressure the patient should be taught to use all parts of the lower lobes. Full expansion cannot be obtained if thoracic joints are limited in range, hence mobilising exercises may be taught, such as easy relaxed movements of the trunk, isolating where possible to the dorsal spine, providing the general condition of the patient is suitable. Once taught these can be advantageously combined with breathing. In addition relaxed movements of head and arms should be included.

Correction of faulty breathing

This again necessitates the use of breathing exercises. The patient is taught to use all parts of the lung, special emphasis being laid on regions which are not being fully exercised. A usual procedure, but one subject to variation, is to train full expiration, then to progress to improving diaphragmatic breathing. When this has been grasped, to teach lower lateral, and posterior costal, and then upper costal breathing. If necessary this is followed by training unilateral breathing. Training must continue until the patient can use any part of either lung at will. It is usually a considerable time before full control of the thorax is gained and, as near as possible, correct breathing becomes a habit.

Correction of posture

Unilateral lung conditions tend to lead to the development of a scoliosis; bilateral conditions to high shoulders, faulty carriage of head, kyphosis and in some cases flat chest and protuberant abdomen. In all cases, owing to disturbance of gaseous interchange and hampered action of the lungs, metabolism is impaired, muscle tone and strength is consequently poor, and the sense of correct posture is lacking. It may be impossible to gain perfect posture, but it can certainly be improved. The patient can be trained to feel what the correct posture is, the postural muscles can be strengthened so that they can hold, without fatigue, a better position and contracted structures may be gently stretched.

Aiding expectoration

In those cases in which cough, due to increased formation of secretions, is present, it is essential to aid their elimination with the least possible strain and effort on the part of the patient. Ineffective coughing is not only tiring, but it results in raised intra-pulmonary pressure and strain on the lung tissue and heart. The patient has, therefore, to be taught to cough effectively.

In cases where mucus is viscid and adherent, percussion on the chest, together with breathing exercises, usually give the patient considerable assistance; if on the other hand secretions have accumulated in cavities or are deep in the small tubes, then 'tipping' should be added.

Improvement of general health

This is mainly in the hands of the physician but some help may be given by use of light general exercises and, where the physician wishes, the administration of artificial sunlight. Improvement of breathing and elimination of stagnant secretions will be followed by improvement of general health.

CHAPTER 2

Acute Respiratory Infections and Pulmonary Tuberculosis

PNEUMONIA IS AN ACUTE inflammation of the interstitial tissue and parenchyma of the lungs. If it is diffuse, involving one or more lobes, it is usually classified as a lobar pneumonia, while if it is localised to scattered lobules throughout one or both lungs it is termed a broncho-pneumonia.

On the whole, though pneumonia may occur at any age, the disease is one which attacks either young or elderly people.

LOBAR PNEUMONIA

In the majority of these cases the organism responsible for the inflammation is one or other of the varietes of pneumococcus, haemophilus influenzae, or staphylococcus. The micro-organisms may reach the lung from the nose and throat by inhalation, or by the blood stream from an infective process elsewhere. Whether or not they actually cause inflammation depends partly on their virulence, but also very largely on the resistance of the patient, which varies with age, general health and the condition of the lungs. The very young and the very old have a low resistance to the pneumococcus, as have those who are undernourished or debilitated. If there is chronic disease of the bronchi or lungs, or congestion due to chronic cardiac disease, the lung tissue will offer a poor resistance to the micro-organisms.

The micro-organisms are usually inhaled into the terminal bronchioles and alveoli at the hilar region, and inflammation starts at this point and spreads peripherally. The pleura is almost always involved in the process and lobar pneumonia is therefore accompanied by pleurisy.

Changes in the lung

The changes are identical with those of all inflammatory processes. The capillaries in the alveolar walls and septa become dilated and congested, consequently inflammatory exudate causes oedema of the walls and interstitial tissue, while much fluid passes into the alveoli driving out the air and causing a state of congestion. The exudate produced as a result of the action of the pneumococcus is typically fibrinous, it therefore clots and the alveoli become filled with a solid substance consisting of fibrin, plasma, red blood cells, leucocytes, lymphocytes and pneumococci. Thus within two or three days of the onset of the condition the lobe is solid, dry and airless—consolidation has occurred.

Before resolution can take place the solid exudate must be softened and this, all being well, is the next stage. Leucocytes, lymphocytes and monocytes tackle the pneumococci ingesting them so that they rapidly disappear, damaged cells are carried away to the bronchial lymph glands by the lymphocytes, while the fibrin is dissolved by the proteolytic enzyme liberated by the damaged leucocytes. Resolution can now occur, because the softened exudate can be removed. Since the pneumococci have been destroyed the blood vessels will return to their normal size, the alveoli will be cleared, partly by coughing up the liquefied exudate, partly by its absorption, and partly by the action of the phagocytes.

If the pleura is involved, it also shows the changes of inflammation. The membrane becomes hyperaemic, and congested, and fibrin is deposited on the surface giving it a rough shaggy appearance. Sometimes a sero-fibrinous effusion occurs into the pleural cavity. The fibrin may organise, and adhesions may bind the two layers of the pleura together.

Signs and symptoms

The patient, early in the attack, complains of severe pain in the area due to the fibrinous pleurisy. This pain is made worse on each inspiration, and consequently an attempt is made to limit respiratory movements of the affected lobe; limitation of movement of the overlying area of the chest is, as a result, often noticeable. To allow fuller expansion of the good lung the patient tends to lie on the affected side.

Cough develops early, at first it is hard, painful and relatively un-productive. Such sputum as there is is stringy, due to the fibrinous nature of the exudate, and rust coloured as a result of the presence of broken down red blood corpuscles. Occasionally bright red blood may be present if acutely dilated capillaries rupture. When softening of exudate takes place copious fluid sputum will be expectorated.

As consolidation occurs, dyspnoea and shallow breathing appear. These are the results of anoxaemia since the exudate in the alveoli prevents the normal gaseous interchange, and possibly owing to toxaemia, the respiratory centre does not react to the increased carbon dioxide in the blood by pro-ducing deeper inspirations. Pyrexia, raised pulse rate and all the signs of acute toxaemia will be present. If there is poor oxygenation of the blood and toxaemia, delirium may occur.

Complications

Many complications may arise, including cardiac failure, as a result of pulmonary congestion and toxaemia, but three particularly concern the physiotherapist—organisation of exudate, abscess formation and empyema.

Organisation of the exudate does sometimes occur though the reason in any one particular case is not always clear. If the fibrinous exudate is not softened reasonably soon, fibroblasts will grow into it from the alveolar walls, followed by capillaries, and this granulation tissue will inevitably become changed into fibrous tissue. Thick strands of fibrous tissue pass from one alveolus to the next and eventually the whole area of lung may become solid and fibrous. This condition is known as unresolved lobar pneumonia and is characterised by persistent cough and diminished movements in the corresponding area of the chest wall.

Abscess formation usually only occurs if the patient's resistance is very low or the micro-organisms are particularly virulent. Actual destruction of tissue then takes place, the alveolar walls break down and a cavity filled with pus is formed. Fibrosis tends to occur in the surrounding area.

Empyema may develop if the patient's resistance is low.

PRINCIPLES OF TREATMENT BY PHYSIOTHERAPY

Treatment by physical measures is not indicated in the acute stage where, as in all acute inflammatory conditions, rest and medical treatment are of prime importance. Since the introduction of sulphapyridine in 1938 and, later, of sulphonamides and broad spectrum antibiotics, patients have recovered more rapidly and fewer require physiotherapy. Physical treatment, however, may be ordered either when resolution is progressing well, or in cases of unresolved pneumonia, or in lung abscess.

RESOLVING LOBAR PNEUMONIA

At this stage the purpose of physiotherapy is threefold: first, to gain full expansion of the affected lobe; second, to improve the general condition and resistance of the lungs; third, to aid the condition of the general musculature.

Expansion of the affected lobe should occur as the alveoli are cleared of the exudate and normal movement should return. Re-expansion is sometimes hampered by pleural adhesions. In addition, through fear of pain, there has been voluntary limitation of movement of this part of the chest and this may continue when pain subsides. For these reasons, breathing exercises are given. The sound side of the chest is steadied by the physio-therapist's hand, while the patient is encouraged to expand the affected area against slight manual resistance. This type of breathing exercise is continued until the expansion equals that of the opposite side.

Improvement of the general condition and resistance of the lung is gained through stimulating the pulmonary circulation by encouraging deep breathing, both expiration and inspiration. Later, when the patient is stronger, trunk movements may be used in addition to the breathing.

The building up of the general strength is an important point because there is a severe degree of toxaemia attendant on pneumonia and the result of illness, even a comparatively short one, is to leave the patient weak and 'shaky'. The general musculature therefore requires strengthening before the patient is allowed to get up. Special attention to all postural muscles is necessary, of particular importance are the back, abdominal muscles and intrinsic and extrinsic muscles of the feet. Careful progression is necessary as the patient must not be tired.

UNRESOLVED LOBAR PNEUMONIA

Physical treatment is very necessary in these cases, since it is essential to try to prevent the formation of fibrous tissue. Therefore, as soon as it is realised that resolution is not proceeding as it should, an attempt is made to clear the exudate and promote movement of the affected area. If necessary postural drainage may be given, but great care must be taken if the general condition of the patient is poor and deep 'tipping' and heavy percussion should be avoided. Unilateral breathing exercises are started at once and given several times a day. As soon as the patient is fit enough, he is taught to give his own manual pressure.

Though unilateral breathing is by far the most important, double-sided expansion exercises should also be given so that general thoracic mobility is improved and circulation aided.

Gradually active exercises are introduced as in the preceding cases.

ABSCESS FORMATION AND EMPYEMA

Though a lung abscess may be the result of lobar pneumonia it more often occurs in broncho-pneumonia, after inhalation of septic material or as a result of septic embolism. Consideration of these conditions will be given later in this chapter.

BRONCHO-PNEUMONIA

Broncho-pneumonia is nearly always secondary to some other condition in adults and children. It may follow whooping cough, measles or one of the other infectious diseases of childhood. Occasionally the inhalation of septic material during operations on the nose, mouth or throat may cause an attack. The condition is very closely associated with bronchiectasis, since plugging of the bronchioles with infected material, and consequently local collapse, is liable to set up an acute inflammatory condition of the small tubes.

It is the lobules rather than the lobes which are affected in this type of pneumonia, and usually lobules scattered throughout one or both lungs. There is an acute inflammation of the walls of the bronchioles with destruction of the epithelium and pus formation. The surrounding alveoli become filled with inflammatory exudate and small areas of consolidation occur. If a bronchiole becomes completely blocked by pus, air cannot enter the alveoli distal to the obstruction, and collapse of the lobule occurs. Thus a characteristic feature of a broncho-pneumonia is the presence of areas of consolidation and areas of collapse. Recovery is very rarely straightforward, it is usually slow with consequently great likelihood of organisation of the exudate with patches of fibrosis. The walls of the bronchioles nearly always show some degree of permanent damage, since destruction of the epithelium is followed by fibrous tissue formation with weakening and dilatation of the tubes.

The signs and symptoms differ from those of lobar pneumonia in that the onset is slower, the temperature rising more slowly but once elevated being more erratic and continuing for much longer. Pain is not usually so marked since the pleura is not necessarily involved if the affected lobules are not near the surface. The sputum is purulent and not rusty-coloured like that of the lobar type. The patient on the whole is more ill and the toxaemia is much more severe since pus is invariably formed.

If physiotherapy is ordered it will follow the same lines as in the preceding type but will be more slowly progressed. Since both lungs have usually been involved bilateral breathing exercises will be used, but very careful observation and palpation will help to decide if any special areas of either side require more detailed attention.

LUNG ABSCESS

An abscess in the lung may complicate either lobar or broncho-pneumonia. It is probably more often the result of the inhalation of a foreign body or some septic material from the upper respiratory tract. Inhalation of such material is not necessarily followed by abscess formation because if the cough reflex is active the substance should be expelled, but there are circumstances where the reflex is depressed. Thus, for example, both morphia and anaesthetics depress the cough reflex, and if substances are inhaled under these conditions they tend to be retained; hence in operations on the mouth, nose or throat under general anaesthesia, there is danger of inhalation and retention of septic material, and consequently of the development of an abscess. Another possible cause is the impaction in a pulmonary vessel of a fragment of a septic embolus from elsewhere in the body; this will readily cause infection of lung tissue.

In nearly every case the abscess forms at the periphery of the lung and lies near either the interlobular or costal surfaces, in these cases the pleura is also very often inflamed. Sometimes the abscess is a closed cavity filled with pus, usually toxic irritation causes proliferation and a fibrous capsule forms around the cavity. Such an abscess is not uncommonly the result of a septic embolus. If the abscess follows broncho-pneumonia or is due to inhalation it more often communicates with a bronchus, though this does not necessarily imply free drainage because the mucosa of the bronchus may be swollen and congested.

According to whether the abscess can drain or not, so symptoms vary. A typical history is that of a rise of temperature and pulse, pain (if the pleura is affected) and a dry unproductive cough. If no communication exists the patient becomes increasingly ill, there is evidence of toxaemia and, in time, marked clubbing of the fingers. In many cases the initial symptoms are followed by the sudden coughing up of a large quantity of greenish-yellow sputum which, if secondarily infected by certain micro-organisms from the mouth, will have a foul odour. The appearance of this sputum indicates that the abscess has now made communication with a bronchus. Should there be really good drainage the condition may undergo spontaneous cure but unfortunately this does not often happen. Usually free drainage is blocked by the inflamed mucous membrane, and general ill-health, toxaemia and cough with expectoration continue. The main object of treatment is to destroy the micro-organisms and to promote free drainage and so gain closure of the abscess cavity. For this reason antibiotic therapy, broncho-scopy and postural drainage are the methods chosen.

Physiotherapy consists of supervising postural drainage. A very careful study of the X-ray film must be made so that a position can be chosen which ensures that the pus will flow from the cavity into the bronchus normally supplying that area. If the pus is thick and does not drain easily percussion to the thorax should be used, though not heavily in the acute stage. Since drainage is so important the patient should take the suitable position every four hours and, where possible lie in the position for half to one hour at a time. It is often considered wise to avoid breathing exercises because on inspiration the effect of the lowered intra-pleural pressure will be to enlarge the abscess cavity. If breathing exercises should be ordered, diaphragmatic breathing only, and with the emphasis on expiration, should be given.

If medical treatment does not prove effective, operative treatment is usually necessary. The most usual procedure is a lobectomy, thus involvement of a larger area of lung tissue is avoided and fear of septic embolism removed. Pre- and post-operative physiotherapy will be necessary to avoid the complications of post-operative collapse of the remaining areas of the affected lung, postural defect and limitation of arm movements.

PLEURISY

Inflammation of the pleura may be a primary condition or secondary to disease of the underlying lung, occasionally it is due to direct spread from neighbouring areas such as the ribs or pericardium.

Three main types of pleurisy may be recognised: dry pleurisy, pleurisy with effusion and empyema. Other cases of pleural effusion exist, but in these cases the effusion is usually the result of mechanical factors, and is not due to inflammation or irritation of the pleura. For example, in both cardiac and renal disease fluid may collect in the pleural cavity.

DRY PLEURISY

A dry pleurisy is a common accompaniment of lobar pneumonia. As a result of irritation, the pleura becomes congested, both parietal and visceral surfaces being involved. Dilatation of the blood vessels results in an exudate which is fibrinous in character, fibrin is therefore deposited on the adjacent surfaces giving them a rough, shaggy appearance. If the fibrin is not rapidly absorbed organisation, by the growth of capillaries and fibroblasts from the pleura, will occur and dense adhesion formation may result, seriously hampering the action of the lung.

Pain, cough, absence of movement of one area of the chest and elevation of temperature, pulse and respiration are features of dry pleurisy. Breathing is painful and shallow because the patient is frightened to take a deep breath. Pain is usually severe and stabbing in type, made worse on coughing and breathing, since on inspiration the tense, inflamed pleura is stretched by the movement of the chest wall. Movement is diminished since it is voluntarily inhibited through fear of pain. Irritation of the visceral layer of the pleura results in a dry painful cough, though expectoration may be present if pleurisy is due to lobar pneumonia.

PLEURISY WITH EFFUSION

An effusion of sero-fibrinous fluid may occur at once or may follow a dry pleurisy after a few days. It is most common when inflammation of the pleura occurs in tuberculosis of the lung, lung abscess, bronchiectasis and pneumonia. Occasionally it follows a primary dry pleurisy when an unsuspected tuberculous lesion of the neighbouring area of lung tissue will be the cause. The fluid may escape into the pleural cavity while quantities of fibrin are deposited on the adjacent surfaces of the pleura. Often the fibrin organises and adhesions form bridging the pleural layers and localising the fluid. If there is much fluid the lung retracts and, if the visceral layer of the pleura is covered with fibrin, it may not be able to re-expand because the fibrotic pleura contracts.

Pain is, in this type of pleurisy, less pronounced because the fluid reduces movement of the ribs and consequently repeated stretching of the pleura is considerably lessened. On the other hand dyspnoea is much more severe as pressure is exerted on the lung. The chest wall may bulge and become immobile due to the accumulaton of fluid, and on percussion over this area a 'flat' note will be heard.

In most cases the fluid will gradually absorb, but there is some danger of deposit and organisation of fibrin with consequent adhesion formation and thickening of the pleura, with limited re-expansion of the lung.

OUTLINE OF TREATMENT BY PHYSIOTHERAPY

Neither type of pleurisy calls for early physiotherapy, particularly if the condition is apparently primary. Medically, both types are best treated by general rest in bed and in some cases local rest of the chest by means of strapping in the position of expiration. If fluid is present, in time, it will usually absorb, and only if it is excessive and causing much loss of aerating surface, or if it fails to absorb over several weeks, is aspiration carried out.

When pleurisy is part of pneumonia, physiotherapy will be carried out as previously indicated for cases of this condition, but if the condition is primary then prolonged rest and, if possible, sanatorium treatment are necessary in order to prevent the suspected lung lesion from becoming active, hence breathing exercises are undesirable.

EMPYEMA

Pus may form in the pleural cavity as a result of direct infection by micro-organisms, or by spread from the lung.

Occasionally a lung, sub-phrenic or liver abscess may rupture into the pleural cavity, or micro-organisms may invade as a result of traumatic conditions of the chest.

One of the commonest conditions to be accompanied by pleurisy is pneumonia. Should an empyema develop during an attack of lobar pneumonia, its onset is usually after the severe stage of the illness, then temperature and pulse unexpectedly rise again; occurring in a case of broncho-pneumonia it usually shows signs during the acute illness. Pus which is streptococcal in origin is thin, and there is little fibrin, consequently few adhesions form. In these cases the pus tends to spread over the whole pleural cavity since it is not localised by adhesions. Pus of pneumococcal origin is usually thick and there is much fibrin, and if the two layers of pleura are in contact, adhesions tend to form which may wall off the pus forming a type of abscess.

On the other hand if the layers are held apart by fluid, a layer of fibrous tissue forms, on the surface of the visceral and parietal pleura, which becomes thick and hard, and as it contracts tends to hamper the movement of the lung and chest wall. Since the pus, in this condition, is contained within a completely closed cavity, the patient will appear, and will be, very ill. There will be a hectic temperature, dyspnoea, pain in the chest, and all the symptoms of toxaemia.

The main object of treatment is to evacuate the pus as soon as possible so that re-expansion of the lung can occur, the empyema cavity is obliterated and dense adhesion and fibrous tissue formation with permanent hampering of respiratory function, is prevented.

Evacuation of pus cannot always be obtained as soon as the condition is diagnosed. The patient may be suffering from a lung affection already, which has seriously reduced his vital capacity, and drainage of the empyema may produce a further and fatal lowering. If the pus is thin and adhesion formation has not occurred, to open the pleural cavity will mean massive collapse of the lung and a shift of the mediastinum. Given time the pus will invariably thicken, and as it thickens adhesions form causing the layers of the pleura to become adherent and the pus to become a localised abscess. For these reasons rib resection may not be undertaken at once, but the patient tided over the intervening period by repeated aspirations and antibiotic therapy.

As soon as loculation of the pus occurs a rib resection is most often carried out, the pus is evacuated and air-tight drainage instituted.

In cases of tuberculous empyema rib resection is not usually carried out. If there is no secondary infection it may be possible to close the empyema by encouraging expansion of the lung. In this case the fluid is drained either by aspirations or pleural wash-outs. If the underlying lung is diseased, and the pleural cavity secondarily infected, it is usual to perform a thoraco-plasty so resting the lung and closing the cavity. Aspiration or intercostal drainage of the empyema may be necessary between the stages of the operation, but drainage is to be avoided where possible because so often a sinus results, the drainage track failing to heal.

Physiotherapy should be started, as soon as drainage is instituted. Its main objects are to gain re-expansion of the collapsed area of lung tissue lying beneath the empyema cavity, to prevent the development of thoracic deformity and to ensure full range of arm movements. Details of this treatment are given in Miss J. E. Cash's book, *Physiotherapy in some Surgical Conditions*.

Occasionally a chronic empyema develops either because drainage has been inadequate or because re-expansion of the lung has proved impossible owing to much thickening of the pleura, or the establishment of a fistula connecting the lung and pleura. In the latter case the suction effect of a negative intrapleural pressure will be lost. In these cases, an attempt may be made to close the empyema cavity either by stripping the thickened pleura or by a modified form of thoracoplasty.

PULMONARY TUBERCULOSIS

Pulmonary tuberculosis is nearly always the result of invasion of the lung by the tubercle bacilli through inhalation either from dried sputum, infected droplets of sputum, or by infected material taken into the mouth. Once inhaled, the bacilli may travel along the bronchi being inhaled from one into another or may be ingested, but not destroyed, by polymorphonuclear leucocytes and carried by them into the lymph spaces.

The reaction of the bronchi and alveoli to the invasion is similar to that of any other tissue. The presence of the bacilli acts as an irritant and provokes an inflammatory reaction. Within a very short time the microorganisms are ingested by leucocytes, which in their turn are absorbed by macrophages. Lymphocytes form a ring round this little mass of cells, their function being to destroy the toxins liberated by the tubercle bacilli.

The complete group of cells form a microscopic cluster known as the tuberculous follicle. Several of these may fuse together to form a nodule about the size of a millet seed and known as the miliary tubercle. These tubercles are avascular and in addition the bacilli produce toxins which cause necrosis of cells, consequently the cells at the centre of the tubercle break down and form a cheesy mass. This process is known as caseation. Subsequently the caseated material nearly always softens. In a great many cases toxic irritation stimulates the fibroblasts to increased activity, and a fibrous capsule forms around the tubercles, in which lime salts are deposited. Healing may then be said to have taken place by fibrosis and calcification.

Whether or not healing occurs depends very largely on the resistance of the patient, and the severity of the invasion, as well as on whether the attack is a primary one or a re-infection.

I

A primary invasion nearly always causes the formation of a small caseous area in any part of the lung, often near the periphery. The bacilli travel in the lymph stream to the hilar lymph glands which consequently become infected. This is known as the primary complex. If the resistance is reasonably high, healing of both caseous patch and lymph glands occurs by fibrosis and calcification. If resistance is low or invasion severe, a rapid spread may occur by the bronchi or blood stream and death ensues.

A second invasion produces rather different reactions. It frequently affects the apex of the lung and evokes an acute reaction. The reaction is characterised by an excessive but localised necrosis of cells, and therefore caseation. The caseated material rapidly softens and, as bronchi are often involved, cavity formation is likely. Spread to hilar lymph glands is very rare. The result of this second infection depends on resistance and type of invasion. If resistance is high, it is possible that the caseated patch may heal by calcification without cavity formation. More often the softened material is coughed up, a fibrous capsule forms around the resultant cavity which is eventually calcified, but a certain amount of infected material may remain in the cavity, and may at some time, if the resistance is lowered, be a source of further trouble, If, on the other hand, resistance is low or invasion occurs in those not previously affected, the process is less localised, the micro-organisms spread and wide-spread cavitation occurs. There appears, in these cases, to be little attempt at fibrosis or calcification. In all cases the pleura over the affected area tends to become involved, thus leading to adhesion formation and thickening of the pleura.

THE PART PLAYED BY PHYSIOTHERAPY IN TREATMENT

The main objects of treatment are to rest the damaged lung, to raise the resistance and so assist the fight against the micro-organisms, and to obtain closure and healing of the cavities. How these objects are fulfilled depends on the severity of the condition, and cases may be roughly grouped into those who require medical treatment, and those for whom some form of thoracic surgery will be necessary eventually. Physical measures are mainly required for the second group, though some little help may be given to the medical cases.

Cases Treated Medically

These patients will include early cases or those who are too advanced to warrant any operative measures. The main treatment for these is rest and long-term antibiotic therapy. Physiotherapy is not usually advocated at this stage, but after the patient has ceased to run an evening temperature resumption of activity is gradually allowed. Then physiotherapy can play a useful part in planning the graduated active work from simple bed exercises, to walking, and eventually to quite strenuous activity. Only in the very later stages are breathing exercises begun, and then they are bilateral with special emphasis on diaphragmatic breathing.

Surgical Cases

Surgery is not used as much today, but for those patients who do not improve with rest treatment, segmental resection or lobectomy may be performed. Should the area involved be too extensive for this form of treatment permanent collapse may be considered provided that the other lung is not too seriously affected. In this case a thoracoplasty performed in stages causes a permanent sinking-in of the chest wall. For all surgical cases pre- and post-operative physiotherapy is essential.

The physiotherapy will be directed at preventing any deformity as a result of the operative procedure, and preventing the accumulation of secretions leading to an atelectasis, following operation. Provided the other lung is unaffected expansion of this may also be encouraged.

CHAPTER 3

Chronic Respiratory Conditions

CHRONIC BRONCHITIS

CHRONIC BRONCHITIS IS a chronic inflammatory condition of the lining membrane of the larger and medium-sized bronchi, usually occurring as a result of infection. It is most common in middle-aged and elderly people, particularly those who live in industrial areas in a cold, damp climate. Occasionally chronic bronchitis may follow repeated acute attacks, but more often it is the result of lowered resistance of the bronchial tree, so that the mucous membrane succumbs easily to bacterial invasion from sources such as the nasal sinuses, antra or tonsils. The lowered resistance may also be the result of some organic change in the lung, such as diminished elasticity which lessens the thoracic movements causing slowing of circulation and stagnation of secretions; alternatively resistance may be lowered by pulmonary congestion due to mitral stenosis or incompetence.

Chronic bronchitis may also be the result of continued irritation of the bronchi by some chemical or mechanical irritant such as gases, dust or smoke.

Pathological changes

As a result of chronic inflammation, hypertrophy of the mucous membrane occurs, the blood vessel walls are thickened and fibrous tissue is formed. The whole lining of the larger tubes usually becomes covered with a viscid mucus. This results in a narrowing of the walls of the tubes and consequently extra strain is thrown on the muscles of respiration if air is to be got in and out of the tubes. If the condition continues unrelieved, degenerative changes occur, atrophy succeeds hypertrophy, the mucous cells, lymphoid tissue and ciliated epithelium are replaced gradually by fibrous tissue; consequently the protective function of the membrane is lost. The degenerative changes tend to spread to the muscular and even to the outer coat, cartilage and muscular tissues become fibrotic.

Signs and symptoms

The outstanding features of chronic bronchitis are cough, dyspnoea and diminished respiratory movements.

The onset is usually insidious. Each winter the patient suffers from a chronic cough, and as the years pass the cough continues for a longer time until eventually it is present the whole year round. This cough is worse at night, disturbing the patient's sleep. Expectoration varies with the state of the bronchial walls. Often the sputum is thin and viscid but when the walls become smooth and atrophic the cough may be quite dry. During acute attacks the sputum is often muco-purulent.

Dyspnoea is always a feature, partly because there is loss of elasticity and therefore diminished expiration and inspiration and partly because the thick mucus hampers air entry and exit into the smaller tubes. These facts mean extra work for the muscles of respiration to overcome the resistance of the inelastic lungs and the narrowed tubes.

In long-standing cases cyanosis may be present. As emphysematous changes occur, pulmonary congestion arises and consequently a greater quantity of reduced haemoglobin is present in the blood stream.

Gradually respiratory movements decrease. Since elasticity is lost, on expiration little recoil occurs. Loss of elastic recoil leads to diminished movements in the thoracic joints. In an attempt to assist breathing, the accessory muscles of respiration are brought into play, the neck and shoulder girdle muscles become tense, and breathing is almost entirely apical. Over-use of the accessory muscles of respiration may give rise to pain in the upper part of the chest.

TREATMENT BY PHYSICAL MEANS

No cure is possible for sufferers from chronic bronchitis but their condition can be improved considerably, and acute attacks can often be warded off. There are four main points in the treatment. Attempts should be made to reduce the thickening of the mucous membrane. This is dealt with by the physician, drugs beings used in an attempt to achieve this object.

The patient must be taught to cough effectively. These patients tend to struggle to clear the tubes by a continuous cough 'high in the throat' without pausing for inspiration. This throws a strain on the heart and vessels and succeeds in making the patient giddy and distressed with no good effect. There are two points to stress therefore. First the patient should breathe in, cough, breathe and cough, and the reason and value of this should be explained. Secondly, the cough must be a deep one, not simply a throat cough; the patient is thus taught to do a short forced expiration.

If mucus is adherent and difficult to cough up percussion is valuable in order to loosen it. There is usually no need to tip the patient and percussion is best done in side lying and lax sitting with the arms and head supported, since both are good positions in which to practise breathing following the percussion.

Control of respiration is most important. Since there is often considerable peri-bronchial fibrosis the lungs are more difficult to move, therefore there is over-use of the intercostals and accessory muscles of respiration and consequently dyspnoea. It is very necessary to train the patient to use the diaphragm more fully, and consciously to relax the intercostals and accessory muscles of respiration. This training must be extensive, since it is not enough to be able to control breathing while in a half lying position or sitting in a chair. The patient must carry this through to all activities, standing and walking in the street, going up stairs, and doing housework. Training may start in half lying and side lying, the patient being taught to sigh the air out of the chest contracting the upper abdominal wall, then after a brief pause to relax the abdominal muscles and let the air be sucked into the chest concentrating on the filling up of the lower part of the lungs. Progression is made to teaching the same exercise while standing, the arms resting on an object such as the back of a chair. The patient is taught to relax the head and shoulders and then practise the breathing so that this can be done if necessary when he is out walking. Further progressions are made in this way.

Training in general relaxation and especially in relaxation of the upper chest are essential since this reduces tension in all muscles and so lessens dyspnoea. In addition it is hoped that there may be associated relaxation of the bronchial muscles. Training should start in half lying and side lying and progress to sitting and even to standing and walking as far as possible. In association with this general correction of posture in the upright position must be undertaken.

Simple easy movements of the neck, shoulders and dorsal spine are an adjunct to the treatment. They are valuable because the chest wall itself tends to become stiff and the posture is poor. They may be done in such a way as to assist relaxation and expiration. Thus relaxed trunk dropping forwards in the sitting position may be combined with breathing and will not only increase movement in the spine and thorax, but will also assist expiration and relaxation.

Another very important point, though one not strictly in the physiotherapist's province, is the *removal of fear and anxiety*. In this the physiotherapist can help by encouraging the patient to talk and stressing the importance of mentioning any fears he has to the physician. If there are home and financial difficulties these should be reported.

EMPHYSEMA

The word emphysema means inflation, and aptly describes a state of the lungs in which the alveoli and alveolar ducts are distended and their walls atrophied. It is a condition which occurs in elderly people, particularly men. A variety of causes may be responsible for the changes, but it is usually associated with chronic bronchitis. There is possibly a hereditary weakness of the lung tissue, and in this case any factor which causes a forcible overdistension of the alveoli may result in permanent dilatation. A chronic cough is therefore a possible cause. A partial obstruction of a bronchus may produce the condition, because, whereas inspiration widens and lengthens the tubes, so tending to overcome the obstruction, expiration produces a diminution in the lumen and consequently increases the obstruction. Air can be drawn into the tubes distal to the partial block, but, once in, it is difficult to expel, and the alveoli become increasingly distended with air. A partial obstruction of this type may be due to chronic bronchitis, or to prolonged attacks of asthma.

An emphysematous condition of part of a lung may be compensatory. If one lobe is removed, the remaining lobes expand and fill up the space in the thorax, the expansion being brought about by the drop in intrapleural pressure consequent to the reduced lung volume.

There is a senile type of emphysema, in which degenerative changes occur in the alveolar walls, but the alveoli are not distended and the lung is small, this therefore is not a true emphysema.

Changes

Continual stretching of the alveolar walls results in atrophy and thinning, and in time the septum separating one alveolus from the next breaks down and disappears. Instead of a great number of alveoli, they are now few but very large in size (see Fig. 4). The intrapleural pressure is reduced, and during expiration becomes greater than atmospheric pressure. This causes the remaining normal elastic lung tissue to collapse, becoming patent once more during inspiration.

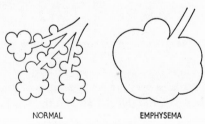

NORMAL   EMPHYSEMA

Fig. 4. Normal and emphysematous alveoli.

Two serious complications arise from this stretching and breakdown. In the first place, the elasticity of the lung is greatly reduced. This means that the lung fails to recoil adequately when the muscles of inspiration relax, therefore the chest wall tends to remain in the position of inspiration. Gradually changes occur in the soft tissues and the shape of the chest alters till it takes on permanently the 'barrel-shaped' appearance in which the antero-posterior diameter equals the transverse, and the intercostal spaces are wider. With diminished recoil of the lung, expiration is decreased, and a greater effort is required to produce both expiration and inspiration. The accessory muscles of respiration are brought into action and dyspnoea develops. In the second place the capillaries in the alveolar walls are stretched, and their lumen diminished, while those in the septa are completely obliterated. Thus the pulmonary capillary bed is markedly reduced, and considerable obstruction to the pulmonary circulation arises. This obstruction results in increased work for the right ventricle, so that hypertrophy follows, and in time evidence of heart failure appears.

Signs and symptoms

The chief clinical signs of the conditions are dyspnoea and cyanosis. At first the patient is dyspnoeic on exertion only, but his capacity for exercise grows less, and he is eventually dyspnoeic even at rest. This dyspnoea is due partly to the difficulty in expiration, the result of loss of elastic recoil

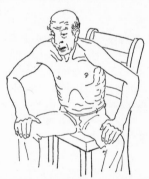

Fig. 5. The usual posture of an emphysematous patient while sitting.

of the lung, which leads to ever greater quantities of residual air and less diffusion of gases between the alveolar air and the blood. It is due also to the extra muscular effort required to move the inelastic lungs and the stiffened thoracic joints.

Congestion in the pulmonary circulation leads to cyanosis since a much greater quantity of reduced haemoglobin will be present in the blood stream.

Cough is not characteristic of emphysema, but as a result of lowered resistance, chronic bronchitis is a common complication, and when this occurs a cough will be present.

The 'barrel-shaped' chest, the kyphotic dorsal spine, the short neck and high shoulders and the diminished chest expansion, are all characteristic features of an advanced emphysema (see Fig. 5).

OUTLINE OF TREATMENT BY PHYSIOTHERAPY

No cure can be expected or obtained, but a certain degree of help can be given to the patient. Treatment aims at preventing recurrent attacks of bronchitis and assisting inspiration by increasing the descent of the diaphragm.

The main object is to increase the power of inspiration making this the active phase of respiration once more, while expiration becomes passive and the intrapleural pressure remains negative (see page 117). Firm pressure is given with the palm of the hand to the abdomen, the fingers spreading upwards towards the costal margin, the patient is taught to 'swell' his abdomen against resistance during inspiration. Just before inspiration ceases the pressure from the hand is eased off, and it is increased just before inspiration starts again. This is progressed by teaching the patient to continue 'swelling' the abdomen during inspiration, gradually removing the resistance.

On no account must he be allowed to force expiration causing 'shut down' of healthy lung tissue but must be encouraged to make maximum use of the remaining lung tissue.

Progression of this work may be practised in altered positions side-lying, sitting, standing and eventually walking on the spot, and then walking maintaining a longer inspiratory phase than expiratory, using manual resistance until the relaxation and breathing become learned, and able to be practised independently.

It should be possible to gain some improvement in the exercise tolerance of these patients, providing the inspiratory breathing becomes a learned pattern and is used all the time.

BRONCHIECTASIS

Bronchiectasis is a condition of dilatation of the bronchi or bronchioles with stagnation of secretions and consequently a tendency to secondary infection and pus formation. The bronchiectasis may be widespread, affecting the tubes of both lungs or all lobes of one lung, or it may be localised to a small number of bronchi possibly in one lobe only. It is found in the lower lobes more commonly, particularly the base of the left lung; possibly because the left bronchus is so placed that it is more readily compressed by any enlargement of mediastinal lymph glands (see Plate X). The dilatations vary in shape; if they occur in the larger bronchi they are often cylindrical, while in the smaller tubes they may be saccular.

Causes

Bronchiectasis may be congenital, but it is much more often the result of obstruction of a large or small bronchus. Such obstruction may be caused by the mechanical pressure of a growing neoplasm or enlarged tuberculous gland. In children the very narrow tubes can be readily obstructed by plugs of mucus during an attack of measles, whooping cough or bronchopneumonia. Immediately following an abdominal or thoracic operation, when secretions are increased and the action of the cilia and the cough reflex are depressed, there is particular danger of the formation of a mucous or muco-purulent plug and obstruction. The air, distal to a completely blocked bronchus, will be gradually absorbed and, therefore, the lobule, segment or lobe will collapse. As a result the traction force of the rib-cage in inspiration will act on the tubes proximal to the block, and these are no longer protected from this force by surrounding air-filled alveoli. The tubes will then tend to dilate, and this tendency will be most marked if they are already weakened by inflammation and infection.

Changes

In early cases, not due to obstruction by infected material, no changes in the epithelium are present. There is simply an area of dilatation surrounded by solid airless lung tissue. Usually, however, there is some degree of chronic inflammation with infiltration of the bronchial walls and surrounding fibrosis. In some cases, sooner or later, secondary infection occurs. Either the original block was formed by septic material, and infection spreads to the walls of the bronchus, or secretions accumulate and become infected. Infection results in a destructive inflammation and the lining is destroyed, the elasticity lost, the wall of the tube weakened so that the dilatation is increased. Infection spreads to the surrounding tissue and fibrosis occurs, and as the fibrotic tissue shrinks further traction is exerted on the tubes. As the walls become increasingly damaged, they lose their sensitivity to the presence of secretions which therefore tend to accumulate, decompose and become purulent. Infection spreads, and cavities may form. On any change of position the purulent material may move and come in contact with healthier mucous membrane, stimulating the cough reflex and so being

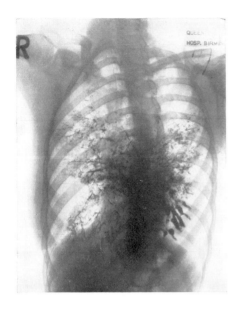
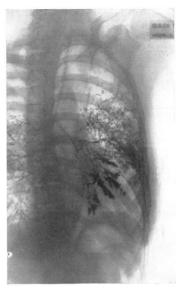

PLATE X. BRONCHIECTASIS (see p. 120)

(a) Showing involvement left lung   (b) Showing involvement middle and lower lobes

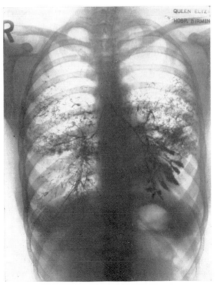

(c) Showing involvement both lungs

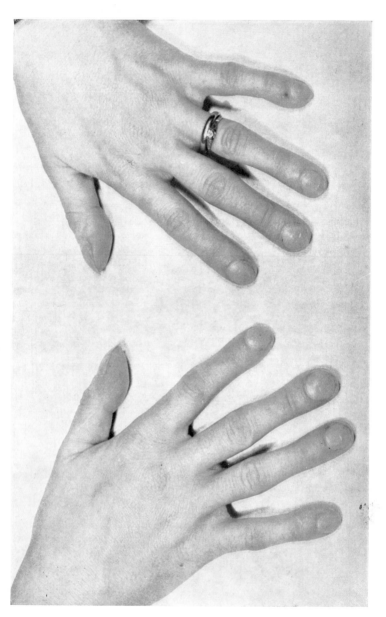

PLATE XI. CLUBBING OF FINGERS IN BRONCHIECTASIS (*see p.* 121)

coughed up. Sometimes the movement is impeded by swelling of the mucous membrane. Pus cannot be drained away then, and there will be toxic absorption, spread of infection and greater danger of the formation of septic emboli.

Signs and symptoms

While there is dilatation and low grade chronic inflammation only, no symptoms may be present, though there is a great liability for recurrent attacks of bronchitis or broncho-pneumonia. From time to time haemoptysis may occur from rupture of vessels in the congested mucous membrane. Once infection is established and pus is formed, cough and offensive sputum are the outstanding signs. Cough is often associated with change of posture since this causes accumulated pus to leave the cavities and come into contact with healthy mucous membrane, so initiating the cough reflex. Sometimes, therefore, the cough is not very noticeable during the day, but is marked on getting up in the morning and on assuming a lying position at night. Turning over in bed may precipitate an attack of coughing, and the patient may find that lying on the affected side lessens coughing, since in this way pus tends to remain in the cavities. The cough may be accompanied by a copious expectoration of foul-smelling sputum, yellowish-green in colour, and the breath then has an offensive odour.

On examination of the chest and the respiratory movements, some flattening of the thoracic wall over the diseased lobe may be noticed and movement may be diminished in this area. Usually vital capacity and chest expansion are decreased.

Since the patient is continuously absorbing toxins and suffering periods of ill-health due to acute bronchitis or broncho-pneumonia, the general health is poor, loss of weight, night sweats, evening pyrexia may be present and clubbing of fingers can sometimes be seen (see Plate XI). Posture is consistently poor.

OUTLINE OF TREATMENT BY PHYSIOTHERAPY

The tendency is for the disease to spread, since toxic absorption and displacement of pus lead to infection of other areas, while plugging of bronchi with subsequent collapse leads to wider dilatation. The constant absorption of toxins is harmful to the patient's general health and resistance, while some danger of pyaemia, and cerebral abscess exists. Therefore the most satisfactory treatment is removal of the affected area or of the affected lobe, but this is not always possible. The younger the patient and the less the symptoms, the better the chances of successful operation. Treatment by physical measures varies according to the nature of medical or surgical treatment.

Non-operative cases

Patients may not be suitable, or may be unwilling to submit to operation. It may be that the condition is too extensive to allow surgical procedures. The object in these cases is to raise the resistance of the lung tissues and keep the cavities as clear of secretions as possible. In this way toxic absorption will be less and attacks of bronchitis may be warded off.

Physical treatment can materially help by means of postural drainage, using percussion and coarse vibrations, breathing exercises and light general exercises. Accurate postural drainage must be carried out at least twice daily, before breakfast and in the evening, for the rest of the patient's life. Consequently it is necessary to teach the patient the correct positions to be used, and how to attain them easily and in comfort at home using available furniture. A careful study is made of the bronchogram, and the drainage positions are chosen accordingly. If no bronchogram is available correct positioning may be carried out by means of choosing the positions and noting those which produce maximum expectoration. Once the positions have been selected they should be tried out, and if they result in little sputum, agility exercises and percussion may be added.

Breathing exercises will relieve breathlessness and assist the circulation to the lungs and bronchi; for this purpose deeper breathing should be encouraged using the chest as a whole. To help loosen pus, localised deeper breathing is taught, particularly encouraging a longer expiration—this breathing being practised best while lying in the drainage position. If the affected lobe is expanding less than the healthy areas, localised pressure expansion exercises are taught, training the patient to give his own pressure either by hand or by strap. Instruction in breathing should not be considered complete until the patient can use any part of either lung at will.

General exercises are chosen to fulfil several purposes. They may be agility exercises to loosen mucus and create slight breathlessness and therefore deeper breathing. Others will be chosen for their effect on posture, and some to maintain the mobility of the thorax and spine. In the case of adults the exercises should not be too heavy and must be well taught so that they can be continued at home. Ideally the patient should receive a course of three or four weeks' treatment and should then continue at home, reporting at intervals of three to six months.

Operative cases

These will usually be children or young adults who have the condition affecting one or two lobes while the remainder of the lung is healthy. A partial or complete lobectomy is the operation of choice though very occasionally a pneumonectomy or thoracoplasty may be necessary. All cases require pre-operative physiotherapy in order to gain the patient's confidence, to drain the cavities so that the lung may be as dry as possible, to establish a sense of good posture, and gain the best possible control of respiration. Physical treatment is necessary again immediately following the operation to prevent collapse of areas of the sound lobes of the affected side, to maintain good posture and full range of arm movements and to gain full expansion of the remaining lobes. (For fuller details of the treatment see Miss J. E. Cash's book, *Physiotherapy in Some Surgical Conditions*.)

BRONCHIAL ASTHMA

The asthmatic patient suffers from recurrent attacks of dyspnoea during which expiration is particularly laboured. The attacks are the result of spasm of the smooth muscle of the bronchi, and swelling of the mucous lining with increased secretion of mucus. These spasmodic changes cause a partial obstruction of the tubes, and consequently extreme difficulty in expiration. Inspiration is not so difficult because, as the chest expands, the smaller bronchi increase in diameter and the obstruction is at least partially overcome but, as on expiration the lungs and thorax recoil and the bronchi decrease in diameter, the obstruction is, if anything, increased. Since air can be drawn in, but not expelled, the alveoli become increasingly distended with air, and dyspnoea and cyanosis result. When spasm ceases, mucus is coughed up, the bronchi relax and breathing becomes normal once again.

These attacks occur most frequently in childhood though sometimes they commence later in life. In many cases no definite cause can be given. It is probable that the broncho-constrictor centre is unusually sensitive and reacts abnormally to stimuli. The centre may then be 'set off' through irritation of the vagal nerve endings by protein substances inhaled or ingested. Such substance may be in the dusts in the house, the coats of animals, or in the factory; it may be the pollen of plants or it may be in certain foods such as eggs, milk, or shell fish. Hypersensitivity to any of these substances triggers off bronchospasm. There may be irritation by the products of bacterial infection in the upper respiratory tract, or the lungs.

In most patients, and particularly when the attacks commence in childhood, there is a strong psychological factor, the centre being abnormally sensitive to psychic stimuli. It has been noted that the attacks occur more often when the home surroundings are uncongenial or there is absence of a stable background. Attacks are more frequent when parents show anxiety in front of the children or when they discuss the attacks before them.

Changes

Changes of muscular spasm and swelling of mucosa are present during the attack but, at first, the chest will return to normal when the attack subsides. Later, however, if the attacks are frequent or of long duration, hypertrophy of the mucous membrane gradually takes place and, in addition, marked thickening of all coats of the smaller bronchi results. These changes serve to make matters more difficult when spasm of the hypertrophied muscle occurs. In time, continued overdistension of the alveoli will lead to atrophy of their walls and areas of emphysema result. Occasionally excessive mucus may plug the smaller tubes and areas of collapse may also be present.

Signs and Symptoms

The attacks come on most frequently during the night but in really severe cases they may occur at any time during the day or night. Sometimes there are premonitory signs, the patient feeling restless and experiencing a sense of constriction in the chest. As the attacks develop and the sense of constriction increases, the patient sits bolt upright and if possible holds on to some object in order to bring the accessory muscles of respiration into play more adequately. Long expiratory efforts are made, interrupted at intervals by short spasmodic inspiratory movements. As more and more air is sucked in and less is expelled, the patient becomes cyanosed, the face is pale and anxious, and the skin sweats profusely. There is wheezing as the air is passed in and out through the excess mucus. The attack usually terminates with a bout of coughing when much fluid sputum is coughed up.

These attacks last a varying length of time, but in some advanced cases, they may continue over several days, the patient, unable to sleep or eat, is exceedingly ill and there is always the possibility of death as a result of the strain on the heart. This state is often spoken of as status asthmaticus.

All patients suffering from asthma, but particularly young children, show defective posture. This is most often a general 'slump' in which the head is poked forward, the dorsal spine is kyphotic, the pelvic tilt increased, producing a lordosis and the chest narrow and flat. Often knock knees and flat feet are seen. This poor posture is probably very largely the result of the mental attitude of fear and anxiety. The anxious child is the child who fails to stand erect to face the world. In addition interference with full oxygenation of the blood leads to imperfect metabolism, and impaired tone and strength of the muscles.

PHYSIOTHERAPY FOR ASTHMA

There is no doubt that much improvement can be gained by the use of physiotherapy, provided this goes hand in hand with other measures. Very little is gained by any treatment if the management of the child at home is unsuitable. Since the physiotherapist is likely to see the parents more frequently than the physician does, she may be asked to reinforce the advice which, without doubt, will have already been given. It is essential that a perfectly normal life should be led. If the child is allowed to consider itself unusual and abnormal, the attacks will be more frequent and a cure is unlikely. Schooling and play should be interrupted as little as possible. The parents should be instructed that under no circumstances should the condition be discussed in front of the child, nor should any anxiety be shown during an attack. If the mother shows anxiety, the child will lose confidence in her, fear will develop and the attacks will be more frequent and prolonged. Once the co-operation of the parents has been gained much can be done for the child. Whether the patient is an adult or a child the principles of treatment are the same, but naturally methods must vary with the age.

Relaxation. To train relaxation is vitally important, particularly in adults who forget the attacks less easily and tend to remain tense and anxious. As in most chest cases, instruction in general relaxation is necessary but particular attention is paid to the muscles of the neck, face, shoulder girdle and chest. Relaxation must be taught between attacks, then, if the patient has premonitory signs, relaxation may be practised and the attack warded off. One of the best methods of gaining relaxation of these areas is by performing relaxed movements. For example, in forearm support, lax sitting, head dropping forwards and sideways and easy rolling are useful movements; in standing the arms may be raised to reach upward and then relaxed, while in sitting the trunk may be dropped forwards. In the adult, attention is drawn throughout to the 'feeling' of relaxation; once the idea is grasped the same relaxation may be gained in sitting up in bed—the position the patient will adopt if during the night she feels an attack coming on.

Diaphragmatic and lateral costal breathing. There is little doubt that in most cases of asthma the ability to use the diaphragm properly and to expand the basal area of the lung is lost. It is almost impossible to perform diaphragmatic breathing if the chest is tense and the neck muscles in vigorous action. The patient has, therefore, to be taught to relax and keep the upper thorax still and to use the diaphragm. Considerable supervision of small children is necessary to ensure that the whole abdomen is not pushed up during inspiration by hollowing the lumbar spine. For this reason, the method of placing a paper boat or tiny shoe on the abdomen and telling the child to let it rise and fall has dangers, it is better to let the patient place the fingers on the area between the diverging costal margins, and to try to swell out round the lower ribs, letting the fingers of the two hands separate gradually. Once the ability to use the diaphragm has been learnt, then the patient may be taught what, in addition to the practice of relaxation, she can do to ward off an attack. It will be explained that provided the diaphragm is used it does not matter how quickly she breathes, consequently she is taught to take the sitting position and practise quick diaphragmatic breathing, so that she can put this into effect in the event of the onset of an attack.

Expiration. Relaxation and diaphragmatic breathing are the two most important measures but an important step is to help the patient to gain a longer expiration so that emphysematous changes do not occur. Attention is drawn to an attempt to reduce the size of the thorax during expiration; once this is mastered then longer expiration may be gained by manual pressure on the thorax. Subsequently, expiration to counting, to the saying of nursery rhymes or to reading may be added. A child will take an interest in seeing how high he can count before pausing to take a breath.

Exercises. Simple exercises will be added gradually, to aid expiration, to mobilise stiff thoracic joints and to improve posture. The latter is most important and a very careful training of posture is required, the methods varying with the age of the patient. Illustrations of such exercises will be found clearly set out in the pamphlet issued by the Asthma Research Council.

Later Treatment

The eventual object of treatment is to gain a good habit of breathing in all daily activities, and to increase the ability to perform exercise producing normal dyspnoea, without provoking an attack of asthma. To fulfil this object the amount of active exercise is gradually increased, while a very close watch is kept on the method of breathing during the activity. In addition, correct breathing is trained during walking, running and climbing stairs, until eventually the patient breathes correctly as a habit. Training begins by teaching diaphragmatic breathing in standing and then while 'marking time'. So many steps are taken on expiration and one or two less on inspiration; this may then be progressed to actual walking, speed being increased till the patient is running, still using diaphragmatic breathing. Walking upstairs may be taken in the same way, beginning slowly three steps up to expiration, one to pause, and two up to inspiration then gaining speed by increasing the number of steps to each expiration and inspiration,

Particularly for children, once diaphragmatic breathing and longer expiration have been taught, class work should be used. This is necessary because these patients can then receive less individual attention with less apparent emphasis on 'asthma', consequently the children enjoy exercises without considering themselves abnormal.

PART IV

Disorders of the Nervous System

CHAPTER 1

Introduction and Clinical Features of Neurological Disorders

REVISED BY ROSEMARY SMITH, M.C.S.P.

DAMAGE MAY OCCUR IN MANY WAYS to any part of the nervous system. Examples are direct trauma or infection, deficiency of blood supply because of thrombosis, mechanical disruption and disorganisation in haemorrhage and in degenerative disease. Lesions of the central nervous sytem (i.e. brain and spinal cord) are irreparable because nerve cells cannot regenerate, and the fibres of the brain and spinal cord have no neurilemma. If the peripheral nervous system is affected, recovery is possible because nerve fibres, which possess a neurilemmal sheath, can regenerate provided their cells of origin are intact. A lesion of part of the brain or spinal cord, however, does not necessarily mean permanent loss of function, for other parts may take over the work of the damaged area to some extent. This is particularly seen in lesions of the cerebral cortex, where quite large lesions in certain areas may apparently cause little in the way of symptoms.

DISTURBANCE OF FUNCTION

The amount of disturbance of function which follows any lesions depends not only on the extent of damage, but also on the mode of onset, the degree of shock, and the particular areas involved.

The mode of onset influences the extent of the disturbance. Sudden onset, such as caused by trauma, embolus or haemorrhage, usually produces more widespread symptoms than will ultimately be present. This is because nerve cells and fibres which were not completely destroyed will recover later. In addition, a sudden lesion is often accompanied by oedema of surrounding tissue and widespread vascular disturbance. In time oedema (causing pressure on healthy tissue) will be absorbed and circulation will be restored to normal. A lesion which occurs insidiously may spread considerably before any marked symptoms appear. A cerebral tumour, for example, may be large before it is discovered.

Sudden and severe damage to the brain or the spinal cord is followed by complete cessation of function of that part of the nervous system. Such a condition is known as cerebral or spinal shock. If the patient lives, some recovery of function will occur. Failure to recover is only present where actual destruction of nerve tissue has taken place. In cases of severe cerebral haemorrhage the patient commonly becomes unconscious, the limbs are flaccid and no voluntary movement is present. If the patient survives, considerable recovery of function can occur. In total transection of the spinal cord, immediately following the trauma, complete loss of all function below the level of lesion is present. In time, however, involuntary movements and tone return, though voluntary movement will never recover.

Some cells and fibres of the nervous system appear to be more readily affected by disease processes than others. The cells of the cerebral cortex degenerate, when deprived of oxygen, in a much shorter time than do those of the spinal cord. The virus producing acute poliomyelitis has a special affinity for the anterior horn cells of the grey matter in the spinal cord, whilst the virus of herpes zoster invades the cells of the posterior nerve root. In peripheral neuritis it is the nerve fibres which are affected, certain disorders involving the motor fibres and others the sensory fibres.

CLINICAL FEATURES

The following clinical features are described because they have a direct bearing on physiotherapy, but it will be appreciated that the clinician in charge of the patient will take note of many more signs and symptoms than are listed here.

Weakness or paralysis
Abnormal muscle tone
Abnormal reflex activity
Involuntary movements
Inco-ordination
Alterations in electrical reactions
Diminished or lost sensation
Paraesthesiae.
Pain

WEAKNESS OR PARALYSIS

A patient is said to be paralysed when he is unable to perform voluntary movement of the affected part of the body. There are, however, two types of paralysis. The muscles will be able to contract if the final common pathway is intact, but the patient may be unable to bring them into action because the ability to initiate and control voluntary movement is lost. On the other hand, the ability to initiate movement may be present but the final common pathway may be damaged and the muscles cannot therefore be stimulated to contract.

In diseases of insidious onset, gradual weakness or dysfunction of one part of the body may be the only feature that a patient has noticed, whilst on examination the clinician may elicit a whole series of other signs of dysfunction showing how much more of the nervous system is already involved. This type of gradual onset presenting with only one or two symptoms is typical of multiple sclerosis, when the patient may only notice the dragging of one foot which starts for no apparent reason and may persist for months or even years before any other symptoms appear.

In diseases of sudden onset such as a cerebro-vascular accident, the initial loss of voluntary movement may be very marked and widespread. However, if the patient survives the catastrophe, there is normally a quick recovery of some voluntary function, further recovery occurring much more slowly.

Voluntary movement may also be inhibited by pain. A good example of this is seen after injuries to the knee, when voluntary contraction of the quadriceps may be lost until the pain is relieved.

Occasionally patients present with an hysterical loss of function of one part of the body or limb. The features of this are that the dysfunction follows no set anatomical pattern, the symptoms may be bizarre, and after full investigation no physical or pathological cause can be found.

Conditions causing weakness may be divided into two main groups, depending on the situation of the lesion in the nervous system:

1. Upper motor neurone lesions, which give spastic paralysis,
2. Lower motor neurone lesions, which give flaccid paralysis.

Spastic paralysis

This is present when there is an inability to initiate voluntary movement although the muscle fibres and final common pathway are intact.

It is now recognised that patterns of movement and not individual muscles are represented in the motor area of the cerebral cortex, and stimulation of this area not only elicits voluntary movement but also the reciprocal inhibition of the antagonists. The nerve impulses travel mainly down the pyramidal tract, but it should be appreciated how closely the pyramidal and extra-pyramidal systems are related and both pathways give rise to excitory and inhibitory fibres.

Most lesions of the upper motor neurone will give a paralysis of this type, which is usually accompanied by alteration in muscle tone. For example, in spastic hemiplegia there is lack of initiation of movement, abnormal muscle tone, and abnormal reflex activity.

Flaccid paralysis

This is caused by individual muscles, or groups of muscles, or bundles of muscle fibres losing their ability to contract. Movement will, therefore, be weakened or lost. The lesion will be found in the final common pathway from the spinal cord. The anterior horn cells from which the axons supplying the affected muscle arise, may be diseased, or the axons themselves damaged so that no nerve impulses can reach the muscle. The virus producing anterior poliomyelitis has an affinity for anterior horn cells and following the acute stage of this illness areas of paralysis will be found, depending on how many anterior horn cells have been attacked.

ABNORMAL MUSCLE TONE

Tone is said to be the state of preparedness of a muscle to respond to stretch. It indicates that the cells of the anterior horn of the spinal cord are in a sufficient state of excitability to be stimulated to discharge if further impulses reach them. This state of excitability is thought to be 'set' by the reticular formation, which itself consists of an excitor and an inhibitor part. Increase in excitability means that fewer stimuli are required to cause the cells to discharge, and a decrease in excitability means the converse.

The reticular formation has an effect on anterior horn cell excitability via a direct connecting link—the reticulo-spinal tract. It is also believed to have a further indirect effect through the muscle spindle. These are specialised organs in muscle which are sensitive to stretch and whose sensitivity to stretch may be altered. These spindles send impulses to the anterior horn cell. In spasticity it seems possible that not only is the anterior horn cell more easily excited, but the muscle spindles are more sensitive to stretch, and thus bombard the anterior horn cell with increased numbers of impulses.

Increased tone

In disorders of the nervous system tone may be increased to the point at which muscles are in a state of tonic contraction, imposing on the patient abnormal postures and preventing isolated movement. This may be due to deficient inhibitor control of the anterior horn cells so that their state of excitability is so increased that they discharge impulses with negligible or fewer than normal stimuli. The increase in tone could also be due to irritation of the excitor reticular formation.

In the former case the inhibitor stimuli may be reduced as a result of damage or disease of the motor areas of the cortex or of the inhibitor part of the reticular formation. This will account for the increase of tone seen in diseases of the pyramidal system illustrated by the spasticity of some cases of hemiplegia and cerebral palsy.

In these cases the spasticity is usually selective and variable. If the anterior horn cells are in a state of increased excitability any afferent stimuli will cause them to discharge, hence slight stretch on a group of muscles, possibly produced by a certain posture, will result in increase in tone in the muscles. In hemiplegia, for example, in the erect posture there is usually increased tone in the flexors of the arm and extensors of the leg. It will be noted that if the muscle is stretched by means of passive movement, tone increases, but if the movement is then arrested or if it is continued until it is nearly completed, spasticity suddenly 'passes off'.

In some cases, probably when the excitor part of the reticular formation is irritated, tone is increased in all groups of muscles of the affected part of the body. This is seen in some cases of paralysis agitans. This type of increase of tone is maintained throughout the whole range of passive movement and to it the term 'rigidity' is applied.

Increase in muscle tone will have a harmful effect on voluntary movement because it acts as a resistance. Moreover, it tends to lead to the development of contractures and deformity and therefore to limitation of range of movement.

Decreased tone

This will result from decreased excitability of the anterior horn cells so that more stimuli are required to cause them to discharge. In certain lesions of the cerebellum, for example, fewer impulses reach the cells through the reticular formation and muscle tone is decreased. Disease or damage of the final common pathway must lead to decreased or lost tone because the cells themselves are damaged or the pathway along which they discharge is no longer intact. Tone will therefore be lost in complete lesions of the peripheral nerves.

Any lesion which diminishes sensory stimuli will result in decreased tone. This will account for the reduced tone seen in tabes dorsalis.

Reduction of tone also interferes with voluntary movement since, on the one hand, a greater number of stimuli are required to initiate the movement and, on the other, guiding and controlling of the movement becomes difficult and inco-ordination is present. In addition, the muscles are less well protected and more readily subjected to trauma.

ABNORMAL REFLEX ACTIVITY

Alteration in reflex activity is a very complicated subject and cannot be dealt with in any detail here. Reflex activity is controlled by higher centres which in some cases actually inhibit, in others damp down and prevent reflexes from becoming excessive. Thus in lesions at cortical level, abnormal reflex activity may occur and abnormal postures, therefore, may be assumed. These may seriously disturb voluntary movement.

In addition, normal reflexes may be exaggerated, diminished or lost.

Exaggerated reflexes

If a reflex such as the familiar knee jerk is unduly brisk, certain possibilities should be considered. It may be because the controlling influence exerted by the cerebral cortex over the reflex centre is decreased or lost and therefore stimuli produce an uncontrolled response. This is the case in lesions of the pyramidal system.

The brisk reflex might be the result of hypotonia in the opposing muscle group. For example, in the case of flaccid paralysis of the hamstring muscles the knee jerk would be exaggerated because, owing to the hypotonic condition, gradual reciprocal lengthening is not shown. On the other hand, reflexes may be exaggerated when the nervous system is intact. Thus in any case where muscle tone is high, as in hysteria, emotional states, hyperthyroidism, deep reflexes will be increased.

Lost or diminished reflexes.

It is clear that any break in the reflex arc, whether anatomical or physiological, will result in lost reflexes. This accounts for the difficulty in obtaining the tendon jerks in tabes dorsalis and for the absent reflexes in a case of cut peripheral nerves or in acute poliomyelitis.

Reflexes will be absent in cerebral or spinal shock though later they may become exaggerated. In cases of general diffuse rigidity, deep reflexes are difficult to obtain because relaxation of antagonistic groups does not easily occur. On the other hand, it must be remembered that most reflexes can be voluntarily inhibited.

Two reflexes commonly met with in cortico-spinal lesions require additional explanation. There is the 'clonus' or repetitive jerk in which, following a sudden stretch, intermittent contractions, at the rate of about seven or eight per second, occur. Increased tone in the particular group of muscles accounts for this. In the case of ankle clonus the calf muscles are stretched, by sharp dorsiflexion of the foot, and respond by contraction. As they relax and the foot swings back the muscles are again stretched and a further contraction occurs. The second is the extensor plantar response, often spoken of as 'Babinski's sign'. Under normal circumstances, except in the infant (in whom the cortico-spinal tracts are not fully myelinated), if the lateral border of the sole of the foot is stroked firmly the great toe flexes.

When the pyramidal system is diseased the great toe extends and in severe cases the other toes fan out and the foot is violently withdrawn. In this case the spinal reflex of withdrawal from the stimulus is no longer inhibited by higher centres.

INVOLUNTARY MOVEMENTS

These are purposeless repetitive movements which may be slow and sinuous, rapid and jerky or sudden reflex contractions. They are usually the result of lesions in the cerebral cortex or corpus striatum.

They need not necessarily be of motor origin. For example, there are reflex spasmodic contractions of muscles which are the result of irritating lesions of sensory nerves.

Examples of involuntary movements which are the result of disease of the motor mechanisms are often seen. There are the cramps and spasms of spastic limbs. These are excited by cutaneous or proprioceptive stimuli acting on spinal areas no longer controlled by higher centres. Choreiform movements are rapid, jerky movements serving no useful purpose. When superimposed on voluntary movement they render the latter incoordinate. These movements appear to be the result of scattered lesions in the cerebral cortex and corpus striatum. Again the student will meet athetoid movements present in a particular type of cerebral palsy. This type of movement differs from the choreic movement because it is slower and sinuous and leads to peculiar positions of joints which could not normally be attained. Such movements are difficult to explain, but are the result of sudden excesses in tone in certain muscle groups and are due to damage to the basal ganglia.

The rhythmic tremor seen in many cases of paralysis agitans is another familiar involuntary movement. The cause of this tremor is uncertain, it may be that it is the result of rigidity. Increased tension of one group causes a slight stretch on the opposite group which is also hypertonic, so a contraction occurs. This in its turn sets up a contraction in the opposing group and so a rhythmic to and fro movement is the result. If the limb is adequately supported so that increased tension in one group does not occur then the tremor may cease.

Fasciculation is another example of involuntary movement. It is the result of irritation of anterior horn cells. In cases of progressive muscular atrophy, for example, these cells are undergoing degenerative changes. Irritation precedes degeneration and so, in muscles not yet showing marked changes, spontaneous contraction of groups of muscle fibres supplied by the axons of these cells is a characteristic feature.

INCO-ORDINATION

Co-ordination might be said to be the ability to perform a smooth purposeful movement with the least possible expenditure of energy. The student will be well aware that to perform even a simple movement at least four groups of muscle must work. These are the prime movers, antagonists, synergists and fixators. Disturbance or improper functioning of any one of these groups leads to inaccuracy of movement and waste of energy. This may be spoken of as inco-ordination.

The correct correlation of these different groups depends upon several factors. First in importance is the cerebral cortex which grades and combines movements to form a more complex action. Second, the cerebellum and corpus striatum are essential. They control the position of the limb, the tone of the muscles taking part, and the rate and regularity of muscular contraction. These sections of the motor system can only produce the right effect if they are kept aware of the position of the body and joints in space, the range of movement performed and the state of contraction of the muscles. The cerebral cortex is kept aware of these things through the kinaesthetic sense, impulses travelling from muscles and joints through the posterior columns of the spinal cord to reach, eventually, the post-central area of the cortex. The cerebellum is informed of these events through the vestibular apparatus and the anterior and posterior spino-cerebellar tracts. In addition to knowledge of position and contraction the cerebellum will only be able to play its part if it is kept in close touch with the cerebral cortex as it will come into action only at the request of the cerebrum.

Even if all these factors are intact, perfect co-ordination cannot be obtained if the final common pathway is diseased, since then messages from cerebrum, cerebellum and corpus striatum cannot reach the muscles. In addition the different groups of muscles needed to perform the movements must be of normal strength and tone (increase or decrease in tone of any one group must inevitably upset co-ordination). Again the presence of involuntary movements may upset co-ordination.

The term 'ataxia' so often applied to inco-ordination should be applied to those types of inco-ordination which are not the result of muscle weakness, spasticity or involuntary movements. If these causes are ruled out two types of inco-ordination stand out: sensory ataxia and ataxia of cerebellar origin.

Sensory ataxia is the ataxia which arises as the result of loss of kinaesthetic sense. The patient, if he cannot see the limb, is unaware of its position in space and so is totally incapable of performing a smooth movement. In addition, muscle tone is reduced since there will be less stimuli from the muscles acting on the anterior horn cells. Co-ordination is, therefore, impaired but is considerably improved if the patient uses his sense of sight as a substitute for kinaesthetic loss. This type of ataxia is present in tumours or injuries of the post-central area of the cerebral cortex, in some cases of subacute combined degeneration of the cord, in the later stages of tabes dorsalis and in many cases of polyneuritis.

Cerebellar ataxia. In this type either because correct messages do not reach the cerebellum or because the cerebellum itself is diseased, inco-ordination is present. If the cerebellum is undergoing a pathological lesion, as, for example, in cerebellar tumour or abscess, or in many cases of disseminated sclerosis, rate and regularity of contraction is impaired and marked hypotonia is present. For these reasons there is inability to steady the trunk or limb, so that during the performance of a movement marked swaying occurs. There is inability to control the movement and so it is carried either too far or not far enough. As the object is approached the movement is not adequately slowed to reach the desired point and so a marked intention tremor develops. This type of inco-ordination is not aided by vision, and this is one of the points which enables the student to distinguish between sensory and cerebellar ataxia.

ALTERATION IN ELECTRICAL REACTIONS

All tissues have certain characteristics of electrical excitability, and the results of stimulation are dependent upon the strength, duration, frequency and rate of change in the intensity of the stimulus, and also upon the state of the tissue itself. The two tissues it is necessary to consider are the muscle and nerve fibres. By means of suitable tests, it is possible to gain information about the state of innervation of muscles and of conductivity in the nerve trunks. Tests of excitability are made by applying a stimulus to the main nerve trunks and to the belly of the muscles and observing the response. These tests fall into two main groups; in the first are the qualitative tests and in the second the quantitative ones.

Qualitative tests. The classical faradic and galvanic tests are qualitative since it is not possible to measure the strength and duration of the stimuli with accuracy. It is, however, a useful guide to the state of innervation of the muscle. The faradic stimulus is an interrupted current of short duration and the galvanic stimulus is a direct current of approximately one second's duration. Where the muscle is normally innervated, a brisk contraction is obtained on stimulating either the nerve trunk or muscle belly with an adequate faradic stimulus. A brisk response is also obtained with the longer stimulus of interrupted galvanism.

With degeneration of the nerve fibres the nerve trunk fails to respond to all stimuli, and conductivity is lost within two or three days of any acute lesions leading to degeneration. The excitability of the muscle itself also changes in degenerative lesions of the motor nerves. It becomes increasingly difficult to elicit a contraction with faradism and, by the second or third week, there may be no response, or only a feeble localised twitch with the maximum current available. Meanwhile the response to galvanism is altering and the contraction becomes sluggish and undulating in character. The loss of nerve conduction and faradic excitability, with a sluggish response to galvanism, is known as the reaction of degeneration and is characteristic of a degenerative lower motor neurone paralysis. If progressive fibrotic changes occur in the denervated muscle the threshold of the galvanic stimulus rises and finally the muscle may become wholly inexcitable, a state known as the complete reaction of degeneration. Massive ischaemic necrosis of muscle leads to an abrupt and early onset of the complete reaction of degeneration.

In lesions where there has only been damage to some of the nerve fibres, the response will differ as some of the fibres will give a normal response while the response from the remainder will be altered. There is a positive response on stimulation of the nerve, the response of the muscle to faradism is weak or absent, and it is sometimes possible to detect both a brisk, and sluggish component in the galvanism. This is termed partial reaction of degeneration.

In recovering lesions it is sometimes possible to elicit contraction of the muscles by stimulation of the nerve trunk before there is evidence of voluntary contraction. On the whole this qualitative test is of little help in detecting signs of recovery.

Strength-duration curve. This test is one of the quantitative methods of assessing excitability, for both intensity and duration of the stimuli can be measured and plotted on a graph. It is desirable to have at least five known selected durations of stimulus. It is found that, as the duration decreases, the strength of the current must increase. In healthy muscle it has been found that the threshold stimulus at one-thousandth of a second duration is in the region of twice the intensity required to elicit a response to a stimulus of one second duration. The differences between the response of healthy and denervated muscle are shown in Fig. 6. Provided a sufficient number of points is available, the graph obtained by testing a partially denervated muscle will show a discontinuity in the curve, i.e. the responses of both innervated and denervated muscle fibres are shown. During reinnervation there are characteristic changes in the responses which gradually become more normal.

Electromyography provides a delicate method of studying changes in electrical potential which are associated with voluntary or involuntary contraction of muscle fibres. The simplest type of apparatus consists of an electrode, amplifier and a loudspeaker. The inclusion of a cathode ray oscilloscope in the circuit makes it possible to observe deflections of the beam produced by the action potentials, as well as to hear the sounds associated with them. Needle or surface electrodes may be used.

As a needle is inserted in healthy muscle, there is a transient outburst of motor-unit activity due to mechanical stimulation of the units through which the needle passes. Otherwise in healthy, resting limb musculature,

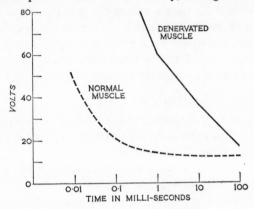

Fig. 6. Strength-duration curve.

there is no detectable activity. Motor-unit action potentials are usually biphasic, associated with a rumbling sound in the loudspeaker, and they are evoked by voluntary effort. The frequency of discharge of any one unit rises as effort increases, and other units are also called into play. During the first two to four weeks after a degenerative lesion, e.g. division of a nerve trunk, the insertion type of motor unit potential may be elicited, but there is no motor-unit activity in response to effort. After about two to three weeks, two types of fibrillation action potential appear; those which are evoked by mechanical stimulation, such as the insertion of the needle electrode, and those which occur spontaneously in sporadic outbursts. They are unrelated to any attempt at voluntary movement and occur rhythmically at rates varying from two to ten per second. In a loudspeaker they give rise to sharp clicking sounds.

Electrical reactions give the earliest reliable information about the presence or absence of a degenerative lower motor neurone lesion, and the first signs of re-innervation of muscle are found by electromyography.

MUSCLE ATROPHY

This is a noticeable feature of many neurological disorders; it is a wasting of the muscle bulk with loss of the typical contour of the muscle. The degree of atrophy is mainly due to the amount of interference to the nerve and blood supply of the muscle.

If muscles are not used to the normal extent, metabolism will be decreased and the muscle fibres will gradually shrink in size. The most pronounced atrophy is seen where there is lower motor neurone paralysis of muscle and no power of contraction remains.

It is not unusual to find that, if the muscle fibres atrophy, the connective tissue framework of the muscle increases in quantity. This tissue has not the properties of muscle fibres and it has a tendency to shorten with the passage of time, consequently the function of the muscle is increasingly impaired. A muscle which is denervated and untreated for a period of one to two years will almost completely degenerate into fibrous tissue.

DIMINISHED OR LOST SENSATION

The disabling effect of diminished or lost sensation depends on the part of the body affected. A slight degree of proprioceptive or cutaneous loss can be very disabling especially in the upper limb.

Damage or disease of any of the sensory transmitting fibres of the central nervous system will result in an interference with normal sensation, depending on the part involved. If, for example, there is damage to the sensory part of the cortex then the part of the body represented in that damaged area will be affected.

In complete lesions of the spinal cord there is a complete loss of sensation below the level of the lesion.

In partial lesions of the spinal cord some forms of sensation only may be lost. In cases of syringomyelia where a spreading lesion occurs, commencing in the centre of the spinal cord, sensations of heat, cold and pain are lost, while others remain intact. Such a condition is spoken of as dissociated anaesthesia, and the actual type of sensation lost depends upon the site of the lesion.

Lesions of peripheral nerves give a varying loss, depending on the nerve. Thus in lesions of nerves which have a large cutaneous distribution there will be a central area of complete anaesthesia, while surrounding this will be an area of partial loss in which tactile loss will be greater than that of pain and thermal sensation. This can be explained by the fact that peripheral nerves in their cutaneous distribution overlap one another, the pain fibres overlapping more than those conveying thermal stimuli.

From a physiotherapist's point of view, loss of sensation is important, and has a direct bearing on treatment. If muscle and joint sense is diminished or lost, inco-ordination of movement must result, though the use of sight, hearing and touch can in part replace the lost kinaesthetic sense. Diminished sensation is dangerous because the patient fails to appreciate harmful stimuli, there is therefore some danger in the application of heat or constant current or any other form of physical treatment in which the patient's appreciation of temperature and pain has to be relied on.

PARAESTHESIAE

Abnormal sensations such as tingling, numbness and 'pins and needles', are complained of in a great number of neurological conditions. These sensations may be spontaneous or they may arise as the result of external stimuli. They are due to disease of any part of the central nervous system and are not always explicable. In some cases such sensations are the result of irritation of sensory nerves such as might occur at the beginning of a progressive degenerative condition—they occur very often, for example, in cases of tabes dorsalis and subacute combined degeneration of the cord. These sensations are not uncommon in partial traumatic lesions of peripheral nerves.

PAIN

Pain is most often the result of irritation of pain nerve endings or of afferent fibres conveying pain sensations. Any harmful agent applied to the skin is likely to stimulate the free nerve endings. Impulses will travel along the rapidly conducting fibres and will be accurately interpreted and localised. This type of pain rapidly subsides. Stimulation of pain nerve endings in deeper tissues is usually produced by pressure or stretching. It is conducted more slowly along smaller fibres, and therefore is insidious in onset and persists longer. This pain is much less well localised. Pain from deep tissues is thus often referred to other structures, sometimes a considerable distance away. The distance to which it can be referred depends on the extent of the area supplied by a segment of the spinal cord. Thus, for example, a lesion in the gluteal muscles may stimulate pain nerve endings so that impulses travel along the afferent nerve fibres to reach the fourth and fifth lumbar and the first sacral segments of the spinal cord. These segments supply an area of skin extending into the thigh, leg and foot, and pain may therefore be felt in any part or all of this area.

It is important to remember that pain may be referred from a distant structure. When a patient complains of pain in the limbs without accompanying signs, careful examination must be made to locate the structure involved. The only treatment which can be successful is that in which the affected structure is dealt with.

L

CHAPTER 2

Examination of Patients Suffering from Disorders of the Nervous System

REVISED BY ROSEMARY SMITH, M.C.S.P.

A DIAGNOSIS OF ALL CASES sent for physiotherapy is supplied by the physician, but before treatment can be started detailed information is necessary as to the condition of the patient and the stage of the disease. This can only be obtained by a thorough examination carried out by the physiotherapist who will be responsible for the treatment. In a case of disseminated sclerosis the diagnosis does not make it clear whether this particular patient shows spasticity or ataxia as the main sign; yet either of these two states is possible and each requires entirely different physical treatment. Correct re-education of recovering muscles in anterior poliomyelitis or peripheral nerve lesions cannot be carried out until an accurate estimate of muscle power has been obtained.

The examination does not need to be a detailed one such as the physician would carry out. It should be directed towards finding out the features of the condition which can be benefited by physical measures, knowledge of which will enable the physiotherapist to give valuable and effective treatment.

It should begin by a brief talk with the patient. Three main objects are gained by this. Firstly, it enables the physiotherapist to make a general observation of the patient while the latter is unaware of this part of the examination. Colour, loss of weight, appearance and manner may all be noted. Secondly, the patient's confidence can usually be gained and his co-operation ensured by a quiet talk. Thirdly, if skilfully conducted, it supplies certain useful data of age, occupation, home conditions and the patient's own history of the onset and nature of the symptoms.

OBSERVATION

Before examining the limbs or individual muscles the patient's posture should be examined in both standing and sitting if the condition allows. A careful note should be made not only of the alignment of that posture but also the contour of the limbs, and the ability or inability to maintain that posture and superimpose an active movement upon it.

Following this the patient's gait should be assessed and any faults in the gait noted, such as steps of unequal length, unequal height or unequal timing, and whether the patient watches his feet as he walks. The tilt of the pelvis on taking a step should be noted, as should the presence or absence of associated arm movements.

The patient, then suitably clothed for an examination, should lie on a plinth or bed in a good light, and in a warm room, so that a more detailed examination may be carried out. Once the patient's shoes have been removed it is often worthwhile to examine the soles of the shoes for any signs of unequal or unusual wear as this will give a guide as to where the patient's weight is being distributed.

Position of the Limbs or Trunk

A close observation should be made of the position in which the head, trunk and limbs are held: any abnormal posture should be noted together with any involuntary movements. For example the hemiplegic patient tends to lie or sit flexed to the affected side. The patient suffering from sciatica holds the hip and knee slightly flexed, while a case of ulnar paralysis shows a partial claw hand.

When the lower limbs are being examined they should first be looked at from the foot of the bed so that they can both be seen in perspective. A check should also be made to see that they are of equal length and girth.

Size of the Muscles

The bulk of a muscle may be decreased (atrophy) or increased (hypertrophy). If atrophy is present examination should be made to discover which muscles are affected. Lesion of a motor nerve results in atrophy of the muscles innervated by this nerve. If a joint is injured or inflamed the muscles acting on this joint will be affected. Sometimes atrophy is the outcome of disuse and in this case a diffuse atrophy will be present affecting all the muscles equally in the area.

If hypertrophy is present there may be an increase in the size of the fibres due to more than normal use or an increase in the connective tissue—a false hypertrophy. The two can easily be distinguished by testing the power of the affected muscles, as true hypertrophy results in increased power, while power is decreased in false hypertrophy.

Any suspected alteration in size should be confirmed by measurement. A point, a definite distance above or below a bony landmark, should be marked on the skin of both limbs. Measurement must be made exactly at this level. A careful record should be kept of the figure obtained on both limbs and the site at which the measurement was made. Difficulty may be met in estimating variations in muscle bulk when both limbs are involved and comparison is therefore difficult. It is worth-while remembering that atrophy causes bony points to become more prominent, also that alterations in size cause alterations in power. The type of individual should also be taken into consideration as the normal size of the muscle groups will tend to correspond with the build and occupation.

Trophic signs

A check should be made on the colour, temperature, texture and smoothness of the skin. The nails should be examined and oedema noted. Changes in these factors may indicate an interruption in the conductivity of sympathetic fibres. Scars and unhealed lesions may be seen. These will occur when superficial sensory loss is added to trophic changes. Lesions then occur because the patient is incapable of feeling pain and healing is slow because the nutrition of the tissues is poor. Poor nutrition to bone will result in the interference with the growth of the bone and may result in limbs of unequal length.

Involuntary movements

Careful watch should be kept for athetoid movements, tremors, muscle spasm and fasciculation. Tremor is usually more marked when the muscles are not actively contracting and the limb is unsupported. Fasciculation occurs most frequently during and after muscle contraction.

PALPATION

Changes in the tissues can often be discovered by palpation. Muscle spasm, increased or decreased tone, contractures, tenderness and variations in limb temperature can all be detected by the sense of touch. For this reason palpation of muscle groups, joints and skin should follow observation.

When the physiotherapist is satisfied that she has discovered all she can by using her sense of sight and touch, tests of motor and sensory function may be carried out.

TEST OF MUSCLE TONE

An examination should be made to see if tone is increased or decreased. If muscle tone is increased a check should be made to see if it is increased to an equal extent in opposing muscles and in all parts of the range of movement, or only in certain muscle groups and specific parts of the range.

If tone is decreased an assessment should be made of the amount of disability in maintaining postures.

TESTING THE STRENGTH OF MUSCLE POWER FOR MOVEMENTS AND POSTURES

It is essential to test the power of muscles both before starting treatment and at regular intervals during the course of treatment so that a record of progress may be made.

Before doing any sort of muscle testing it is important that the patient should be warm and in a comfortable position and it is more satisfactory if the same physiotherapist who does the initial testing should do the succeeding ones.

Muscle power for active movement may simply and effectively be tested by the numerical scale suggested by the Medical Research Council. The scale is as follows:

    o = no contraction
    1 = flicker, but no actual movement
    2 = contraction producing movement when gravity is eliminated
    3 = contraction against the force of gravity
    4 = contraction against gravity and some resistance
    5 = normal strength

Descriptions of the technique are to be found both in the Medical Research Council's handbook and in Kendall and Kendall (1949). By recording the results of the test on a chart, the patient's progress can be seen at a glance (see Fig. 7, p. 148).

The strength of muscle power for maintaining postures including static work in all parts of the range of movement should be assessed. Unless the patient can maintain a certain posture it is impossible for him to superimpose a voluntary movement upon it.

An observation should be made of the patterns of movements and postures, and if they are abnormal they may be assessed by the neurological assessment chart first correlated by Mrs Bobath. The chart is also from o–5 and is assessed as follows:

    o = patient cannot be put into position
    1 = can be put into position passively, cannot hold it, or cannot be left
    2 = can be placed, can hold it
    3 = patient can take the position actively, it is abnormal
    4 = patient can take the position actively without any help, it is nearly normal
    5 = normal

A functional activity chart should also be made and this is usually done in co-operation with the occupational therapy department and ideally combines a home visit, so that a complete picture can be made of the patient's main disabilities in regard to everyday activities (see Part VII: The Management of Physical Disability, page 271 et seq.).

FACSIMILE OF PROGRESS CHART OF A PATIENT WITH A RADIAL NERVE INJURY

NAME: A.............................. R..............................

Dates	5.vii 1951	19.vii	2.viii	16.viii	12.ix	10.x	21.xi	16.i 1952	30.iv	29.x
Types of Contraction	Voluntary									
Brachioradialis	2+	4	4	4+	4+	5−				
E. C. Rad. L.	2	3+	4	4+	4+	5−	?5	5	5	5
E. C. Rad. B.	?1	?3	4−	4+	4+	5−				
Sulpinator										
E. D.	?1	2+	3+	4−	4−	4	4	4	5−	5
E. D. Min.	0	0		?	?	?2	?4	4	4	?5
E. C. Uln.	0	2+	3+	4	4+	4+	?5	4+	5	5
Abd. P. L.	0	0	2+	3	3+	4	4+	4+	4+	4+
E. P. L.	0		2	3	3	3+	4	4	4	5
E. P. B.	0		?1	1	3	3+	3+	4	4	5?
E. Indic.	0		0	0	0	1	3	?3+	4	4
Ner Conduction: Elbow										

Charts are available for different groups and for the upper and lower limb plexuses. In the columns provided, the response to galvanism and faradism can be indicated for each muscle. In this case, voluntary testing only is recorded.

Fig. 7

At this point it is worth remembering that although a patient may have a long list of motor and sensory symptoms the fact that she cannot for example lift a kettle from the stove or put her stockings on will be of prime importance to her, and if she can be helped over these domestic hurdles she will benefit greatly and consequently co-operate to the full.

ELECTRICAL TESTS

These should be carried out where there is true muscle weakness or paralysis. It is important to warm the muscles before starting any test so that they can function at their best. If there is no nerve involvement the reactions to stimulation with faradism and with interrupted galvanism will be found to be normal. A comparison should be made with a normal muscle, preferably the same muscle on the other side of the body. A weak normal response is an indication that, although all the nerves are intact, the muscle fibres are atrophied and are, therefore, not contracting with their usual strength. A sluggish response to interrupted galvanism is an indication that there are at least some denervated fibres in the muscle. If this is accompanied by no response to faradism a complete reaction of degeneration is present showing that the muscle has no nerve supply. If, however, it is found that the sluggish galvanic response partners a weak contraction to the faradic current is can be assumed that only some of the nerve fibres are missing and a partial reaction of degeneration is present.

If the strength-duration curve is the method chosen, the curve obtained from the paralysed muscle will be found to be quite different from the normal curve. The two curves can be plotted on graph paper, and the difference between them noted. If regular tests are taken it will be seen that as the affected muscle improves the strength-duration curve will gradually alter its shape returning towards the normal.

The most accurate method of carrying out an electrical test is to record the electrical impulses actually arising from the affected muscle. This is called an electromyograph and is only carried out by an experienced physician. When making electrical tests it should always be remembered that degeneration of nerve tissue, following an injury, is not complete for at least ten days, and no reliable record can be obtained until after that time has elapsed.

TESTING RANGE OF MOVEMENT

Range of movement is tested by moving the joint passively in all the directions that the particular joint allows. It may be limited by many factors. In neurological conditions limitation is most commonly the result of either degenerative changes in joints due to disturbed circulation and disuse, or adaptive shortening of muscles and tendons occurring as a result of spasticity or flaccidity of muscle. If the muscles are hypertonic, limitation of range indicates that spasticity is severe; if hypotonic then joints can be carried beyond their normal range. In both cases it is important to appreciate that it is the length of the muscles that is being tested, therefore a muscle passing over two joints, such as gastrocnemius, needs special testing.

Contractures in fascia and capsule can occur especially when the sympathetic nervous system is involved.

TESTING CO-ORDINATION

It is essential for the physiotherapist to be aware of the presence of inco-ordination. It is also necessary to know the cause of this condition, as the method of re-education varies with the cause. The way in which the patient performs the active movement used in the examination of muscle power is carefully watched. Special tests are also given—these may be selected as desired but usual tests are: placing the heel of one foot on the patella of the other leg, or touching the examiner's finger with the patient's finger.

In order to decide whether the faulty movement is due to kinaesthetic loss, or to lesions of cerebellar tracts or cerebellum, the patient should first perform the movement with the eyes open and then with the eyes shut. Any discrepancy should be noted. The type of inco-ordination may also be recognised by noticing other points; does the patient eventually reach his object? Is there a side to side deviation as the object is neared (an intention tremor)? Does the proximal segment of the limb sway as the movement is performed? If all these points are present the lesion is probably cerebellar.

TESTING SENSATION

It is not necessary to carry out a full examination of the sensory system but it is essential for the physiotherapist to be aware of the loss of sensations of pain, temperature and position. Thermal sense should be tested by lightly touching the skin with hot and cold test tubes. The test should be commenced on normal skin and move gradually on to the part to be tested. It should also be compared with the normal side. The patient's eyes should be screened throughout the test. Pain sensation is tested by pin-prick in a similar fashion. In each case speed and accuracy of response should be noted.

Examination of the sense of position of joints should be carried out with the eyes closed and the joints are moved passively into different positions and the patient is asked to state what position he thinks the joint to be in.

As with the recognised tests for co-ordination care should be taken not to include these simple tests in any treatment session as they would obviously lose their value as tests.

It is clear that the foregoing detailed examination cannot be carried out in one session and if the patient does require such a detailed examination this may be carried out over several days or even weeks.

CHAPTER 3

Principles of Treatment of Neurological Disorders by Physiotherapy

REVISED BY ROSEMARY SMITH, M.C.S.P.

THE MAIN AIM OF TREATMENT for a patient suffering from a neurological disorder is to make him as independent as possible within his limits. Treatment is directed from the beginning both to the affected muscle to assist recovery and prevent contractures and to the hypertrophy and re-education of normal muscles.

Completely destroyed nervous tissue in the brain and spinal cord cannot regenerate, but even after severe trauma within the central nervous system some recovery of function usually occurs, due to one or more of the following factors:

1. Relief of pressure.
2. Hypertrophy of remaining innervated muscle.
3. Stimulation of inactive neurones.
4. Hypertrophy of unaffected muscles.

RELIEF OF PRESSURE

A vascular or inflammatory lesion may not only destroy cells but may result in widespread haemorrhage and oedema causing pressure on nerve cells and fibres, thus putting them out of action for a period of time. Within a few weeks of such a catastrophe oedema begins to subside as fluid is absorbed into the blood and lymph stream. Those cells which have not been permanently damaged are gradually released from pressure and may begin to resume function. This fact accounts for the extensive recovery of paralysed muscles within the first few weeks following an attack of acute anterior poliomyelitis. All the recovery which will result from this absorption of oedema will probably occur during the first six weeks; any recovery which occurs after this will be due to other factors.

Physiotherapy cannot assist this absorption and recovery.

HYPERTROPHY OF REMAINING INNERVATED MUSCLES FIBRES

The strength of a muscle contraction depends on the number of motor units stimulated, also the frequency of impulses down the motor neurone.

The motor unit which consists of an anterior horn cell, motor fibre, myoneural junction and the hundred or more muscle fibres, obeys the all-or-none law which is to respond maximally to stimulation or not at all. However, in severe fatigue or disease some muscle fibres stop contracting and rest, and then join in again and so do not absolutely obey the all-or-none law. The motor unit is influenced by the level of excitation of the anterior horn cell resulting from proprioceptive and postural reflexes and afferent discharges from the cerebellum, basal ganglia and brain stem. Even in a normal person the anterior horn cells vary in excitability and have different thresholds of excitation.

It is the activity of motor units which results in therapeutic benefit to a muscle in the form of hypertrophy. Only after application of maximal resistance do a greater number of motor units respond, the aim of treatment therefore is to stimulate the maximum number of anterior horn cells within the spinal cord which will in turn excite the greatest number of motor units in a paresed muscle.

Any techniques which can produce this result may be used, the important factor being to employ the simplest form of exercise which will produce the greatest therapeutic benefit to the muscles.

All forms of resisted exercise including gravity resisted, dead weight resisted and spring resisted exercise, obviously have a place here as do water resisted exercises if these are available.

The use of proprioceptive facilitation techniques are of great benefit if applied simply and correctly, bearing in mind that each patient presents a different problem and no rigid pattern can be universally applied. By adding facilitation to maximal resistance a greater response in paresed muscle can be demonstrated. For example it can be shown that a muscle which fails to respond to a free voluntary movement can respond to the application of stretch, maximum manual resistance and a mass movement pattern, e.g. extension and abduction of the hip. Thus facilitation was necessary to raise the level of excitation within the central nervous system above threshold, and cause some hitherto dormant anterior horn cells to discharge.

A programme of facilitation techniques is applied directly to the central nervous system and thus indirectly to the muscles. All the techniques increase central excitation and thereby enhance voluntary activity in paresed muscles.

STIMULATION OF INACTIVE NEURONES

In the central nervous system there are many more neurones than are actually in everyday use. Following trauma or disease within the central nervous system these hitherto dormant neurones may be trained to take over the function of the now inactive ones. Because of their higher threshold of excitation strong sensory stimulation is needed to excite them and thus establish new pathways within the central nervous system.

Proprioceptive neuromuscular facilitation techniques can be used to increase the level of excitation within the central nervous system and thus establish new pathways for the transmission of voluntary impulses.

A broad outline of the technique of proprioceptive neuromuscular facilitation now follows. The student must of course be aware that their application is not confined to neurological disorders and they are incorporated in a wide variety of treatments where re-education of movement and posture is required.

The techniques were first described by Dr Herman Kabat and his associates, working in the field of neuromuscular physiology and applying it to physical medicine.

Maximal Resistance

Resistance increases excitation within the central nervous sytem, and therefore the voluntary response of the muscles. Because of the increased tension in muscles and related structures, there are increased afferent proprioceptive impulses, which serve to facilitate voluntary response in the muscle by lowering the threshold of excitation of the anterior horn cell.

Maximal manual resistance is used in all techniques of proprioceptive neuromuscular facilitation and the position of the physiotherapist's hands giving resistance should be such that they adequately control the desired movement and lie in the direction of the movement.

The value of manual resistance is twofold. Firstly it stimulates cutaneous nerves; and secondly it can be varied to match the patient's muscle power, and so an active contraction can occur throughout the whole range of movement or be localised to part of the range as desired.

Mass Movement Patterns

A single muscle or an isolated movement is hardly ever used in voluntary activity. Normal voluntary movement is characterized by related muscle groups working together and the harder a particular group is made to work the more associated muscles are brought into play. This spread of excitation within the central nervous system into functionally related muscle groups is known as irradiation.

Facilitation can be achieved by the use of a mass movement pattern of a whole limb against resistance; normal muscles in the pattern respond with sufficient power to cause overflow of excitation within the central nervous system to innervate the paresed component.

Spiral mass movement patterns are more effective than straight ones because of the diagonal distribution of muscles. Stretch and maximum resistance are applied to all mass movement patterns.

Even greater facilitation may be achieved by using reciprocal mass movement patterns of the upper or lower extremity. For example, the response of a paresed muscle in the lower limb may be augmented by a combination of mass movement patterns of the leg with the opposite stronger arm.

Mass movement patterns need not always be taken through their full range and in some cases hardly any range is permitted to gain irradiation into a particular group. Irradiation can occur from functioning proximal muscles to paresed distal ones or vice versa.

It must be remembered that it is not the patterns of movement themselves that are being re-educated but the patterns are being used to facilitate dormant nerve cells. Versatility is the key to success in using these techniques.

The following diagrams in Fig. 8 show the basic diagonal mass movement patterns of the upper and lower extremity.

Successive Induction

This is the facilitation which one reflex exerts on another.

The physiologist Sherrington demonstrated that immediately following flexion the excitability of the extension reflex was greatly increased. In most daily activities antagonist movement immediately precedes the main agonist movement, so by applying resistance to the antagonist in preparation for a resisted movement of the agonist there is an increased contraction of the antagonist and therefore greater facilitation to the agonist.

This axiom can be made use of for facilitation purposes when one antagonist group is much stronger than the other. For example, with a weak triceps and a strong biceps, a strong contraction of the biceps against resistance followed by a resisted contraction of the triceps results in a greater, facilitated, contraction of the triceps.

It is at once obvious that the first contraction must be of the stronger group.

If the imbalance between two opposing muscle groups is extreme this use of successive induction, which is called reversal of antagonists, has to be restricted as there is danger in increasing the imbalance.

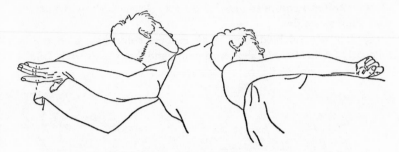

Fig. 8. A. Diagonal spiral pattern: upper extremity. Manual resistance of therapist is in direction opposite to that of motion of patient in this and the diagonal patterns of the following figures.

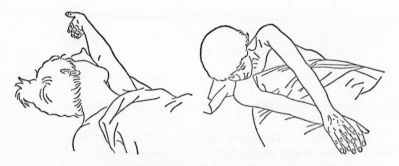

Fig. 8. B. Diagonal spiral patterns: upper trunk.

(Figure 8 is taken from Chap. XIII of *Therapeutic Exercise*, with the permission of the author, Dr. Herman Kabat and Elizabeth Licht, publisher, Newhaven.)

Reversal of antagonists can be used for facilitation techniques in three different ways:

(i) Slow reversal of antagonists—this is alternating isotonic contractions of two antagonist groups of muscles against resistance, always contracting the strong group first.

(ii) Slow reversal hold—this is an isotonic contraction of one group followed by a 'hold' in the shortened range, and then immediately followed by the same isotonic and 'hold' contraction in the opposing weak groups.

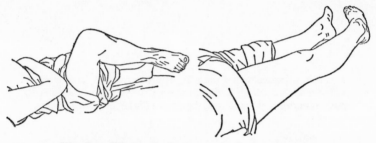

Fig. 8. c. Diagonal spiral pattern: lower extremity.

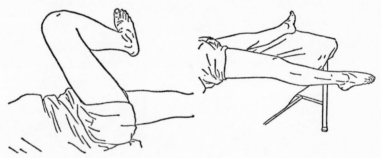

Fig. 8. D. Diagonal spiral pattern: lower extremity.

(iii) Rhythmic stabilization—this is repeated 'isometric' contractions of two antagonist groups of muscles against resistance which allows no range of movement in the joint, but may be performed in all parts of the range of movement for that joint. Once again the strong group is contracted first.

It must be remembered that the word isometric now has no literal meaning, for although the muscle may appear not to change in length the contractile element of the muscle must shorten when contraction occurs. However, the elastic element compensates for this shortening thus making the muscle appear unchanged in length.

REFLEXES

Various proprioceptive reflexes can be used to reinforce voluntary effort. The simplest one is the stretch reflex.

Stretch applied to a paresed muscle elicits a stronger response, and maximum response from stretch will be obtained by putting not only the prime mover but also the related muscle groups in their fully stretched position. By stimulating the stretch reflex and voluntary movement in the same muscle at the same time the reflex excitation may be used to stimulate the voluntary movement.

The Von Bechterew reflex is mass flexion of the lower extremity, stimulated by flexion of the great toe; this may be stimulated at the same time as the patient attempts voluntary flexion of the lower extremity, and a greater response will be elicited.

The positive supporting reflex is an extensor reflex, induced by pressure on the plantar surface of the foot; this can be used to facilitate a voluntary thrust of the lower limb.

Righting reflexes can be used to facilitate voluntary movement in techniques of resistive balancing. This can be done in various starting positions i.e. standing, sitting, or kneeling, and the patient is pushed slowly in various directions in an attempt to throw him off balance. The righting reflexes thus facilitate the various muscle groups involved in maintaining posture.

Defective balance is found in both upper and lower motor neurone disease and may be due to muscle weakness, abnormal tone, defective sensation or contractures, as well as in cases where there is involvement of the vestibular part of the ear or brain stem.

Use of eyes and ears. Anterior horn cells are also stimulated through pathways from the eyes and ears. Thus, if maximal bombardment of motor cells is required to bring into action all available motor units, the patient must be encouraged to watch what he is doing and the physiotherapist must make use of her voice to give emphatic commands.

Use of volition. Motor cells are normally excited through pathways from motor centres in the cerebral cortex. These pathways are rarely completely destroyed and should be used to their maximal capacity. The patient should make a strong effort to think of each movement throughout the treatment.

HYPERTROPHY OF UNAFFECTED MUSCLES

If a lesion in the central nervous system is complete and no further recovery seems possible, then other muscles or muscle groups must be trained to restore as much independence as possible to the patient. When a patient has a permanent disability the unaffected muscles should be developed to their maximum strength.

If for example there is a complete lesion of the spinal cord at T. 10, treatment is directed as much to the normal as to the denervated muscle groups. Muscles with a high nerve supply spanning a large area, such as latissimus dorsi (C. 5.6.7.) can, by working from reversed attachments, assist the patient in lifting the pelvis, thus clearing the foot off the ground in walking.

In more localised lesions where perhaps one vital muscle is not functioning, surgery may be employed to transplant a healthy functioning muscle tendon to do the work of the paralysed one, and this must consequently be re-educated to take over its new function.

FACTORS HAMPERING RECOVERY

Some recovery of voluntary power and independence in neurological disorders may well occur through one or more of the ways previously indicated but such recovery is often hampered by abnormal muscle tone, by the development of contractures and deformity, by stiff joints, by impaired circulation and by pain. These, therefore, require treatment or prevention.

ABNORMAL MUSCLE TONE

Some tone in muscles is necessary for the maintenance of posture and the performance of movement. If tone is excessive it is difficult for prime movers to overcome the resistance offered by hypertonic muscles. If tone is too low, then the guiding and controlling of the movement becomes reduced or lost. In both cases movement, if present at all, becomes incoordinate.

Increase in tone is usually the result of lack of inhibitory control by higher centres and it results, if it is permanent, in typical postures, and absence or abnormalities of voluntary movement. Such movements as occur are largely of the reflex type, that is, on attempted movement there is simultaneous contraction of all the muscles of one type of pattern. Thus on attempting to extend the fingers, flexion of the wrist and elbow with pronation of the forearm and abduction of the shoulder occurs.

Treatment is aimed at relaxing muscle tone, followed immediately by re-education of voluntary movement, as weakness in antagonist muscle groups is a constant finding due to disuse. The following methods may be employed.

(i) Relaxation techniques based on the laws of successive induction and reciprocal innervation. These laws were first described by Sherrington, when he stated that stimulation of an end-organ in the agonist caused cessation of impulses along the motor neurone to the antagonist. However, all his observations were made on decerebrate and anaesthetised animals, therefore not under voluntary control. He did say that antagonists could contract together but called this double reciprocal innervation in which the balance of inhibitory and excitory impulses was such as to allow both half centres to discharge.

Later, Tilney and Pike rejected Sherrington's theory, saying that muscular co-ordination depends primarily on synchronous co-contractive relation of antagonists. Inactivity of the antagonist is not synchronous with inhibition. The difference in the observations is explained if volition is taken as the modifier of the reflex state. However, in spasticity which simulates decerebrate rigidity more closely, reciprocal innervation is a constant finding. Thus, during contraction of the agonist, relaxation of the spastic antagonist does occur. The technique is applied thus: the spastic group is placed in a fully stretched position and the patient asked to attempt a voluntary contraction of the group against maximum resistance, and no range of movement is allowed. The patient is then asked to relax the spastic group and this is followed immediately by an active contraction of the weak antagonist group against resistance. The greater the contraction of the spastic group the greater will be the contraction of the antagonist group by successive induction, and the greater the contraction on the antagonist the greater will be the relaxation in the spastic group by reciprocal innervation. Isotonic contractions tend to increase spasticity whilst 'isometric' contractions tend to decrease it.

(ii) Application of ice packs to spastic limbs. As spasticity is the result of hyperactive reflex activity it can be shown that the effect of cold is to cause reflex relaxation. It will be remembered that there are afferents to the anterior horn cells from the sensory nerve endings in the skin, so by stimulating them, one reflex is used to inhibit another. The method and time of application of ice packs to spastic limbs is related to the patients' tolerance and also to the degree of spasticity. Care should be taken to enquire whether the patient has a previous history of sudden fainting or collapse which may be due to vasovagal or emotional causes, but producing a rapid lowering of the blood pressure. These patients should only have ice packs applied under strict supervision.

Immediately following the application of ice, the muscles should be re-educated in their increased length.

(iii) Reflex inhibition in posture and movement. These techniques which were developed by Bobath, are described in the chapter on cerebral palsy, p. 189.

M

Decrease in tone. This causes ataxia, and may be seen in many cases of disseminated sclerosis. The patient is able to perform voluntary movement but this is inco-ordinate because there is insufficient postural fixation and because of intention tremor. For example, there may be ability to move the arms but the patient cannot feed himself because swaying and intention tremor make it impossible to get the food into his mouth.

It will be remembered that the decrease in tone resulting in ataxia may be due to decrease of sensory stimuli flowing into the central nervous system or it may be due to lesions in the cerebellar system. If the former is the cause, the main object is to increase the sensory stimuli reaching the motor centres. Hence, once more, use is made of alternative pathways and activation of 'dormant' neurones. The patient is trained to see, feel and hear what he is doing. Simple movements are repeated time after time so that synaptic resistance is reduced in the pathways which are still available. Movements are performed in such a position that the patient can watch every step. When possible they are carried out on a firm surface so that a greater amount of sensory stimulation is produced. They are often done in time to counting so that the patient 'hears' the movement. In walking a stick may be used to tap the ground evenly before the feet are brought down, for the same reason.

If the lesion is in the cerebellar system the principle is again the development of inactive but unaffected neurones and the establishment of alternative pathways. Volition is particularly important; the patient must concentrate on what he is doing and make a supreme effort to control the movement. Simple movements are taken and are repeated time after time. The movement is stopped and begun again if any jerk occurs.

In this way maximum stimulation of cerebellar and anterior horn cells will occur.

Facilitatory techniques may also be used for this purpose. Reversal of antagonists often proves most successful in gaining balance control. For example the patient may be unsteady in sitting. He is then instructed to try to prevent the physiotherapist pushing him first in one direction and then in the other. This is repeated constantly and balance tends to become steadier due to the increase in strength of opposing muscle groups. Resistance also may be used because it increases the sensory stimuli reaching the cerebellum from muscles and joints.

CONTRACTURES AND DEFORMITIES

Deformities tend to develop in pyramidal and lower motor neurone lesions, in striatal damage and in children showing circulatory disturbances. They are the result of adaptive contractures where there is muscle imbalance, of contracture of fibrosed joint structures following oedema, or of impairment of growth. It is essential that they should be prevented or they will hamper such recovery of voluntary power as is possible. Splinting, passive movements, massage and elevation to relieve oedema and strengthening of weak muscles are the methods of choice.

Splinting is valuable because it maintains a good position and prevents contractures, or provides a continuous stretching force if contractures have already commenced.

When splints are used, therefore, certain rules should be observed. They must fit perfectly and all 'pressure points' must be protected. They must be removable so that joints may be carried through their full range daily, and the skin toilet attended to. In growing children the splints must be checked frequently so that they are always the correct fit. They must be light so that they add no more weight than is necessary to a weakened limb, and they must be of material which will stand up to wear and tear. They should be easy to apply so that they can be taken off at home and re-applied correctly.

Where possible, splints should allow movement of the joint but return it to its correct position, that is, a splint should stimulate the action of the paralysed muscles. Such splints are known as 'lively' splints.

STIFF JOINTS

If joints become stiff the recovery of voluntary movements is severely hampered. Treatment should be directed from the beginning to avoid stiffness in joints and full range should be assisted. Active movements must be frequently and thoroughly performed. If the joints have become stiff the following relaxation technique may be applied if the patient's physical condition allows it. It is combined with the use of an ice pack placed on the tightened structure. The limb is put as far as possible into the shortened range, then a resisted contraction of the antagonist allowing no range, then a resisted contraction of the agonist combined with slight over-pressure from the physiotherapist plus a 'hold' contraction in the shortened position. Then the command to relax and, without allowing the patient to lose any of the range gained by the previous contraction, begin the technique again.

ATROPHY OF MUSCLES

Lack of normal use inevitably results in muscle atrophy and, consequently, as voluntary movement becomes possible, recovery is hampered by loss of power. Atrophy is at least partly prevented by all the steps taken to regain voluntary power. In cases in which there is paralysis of muscles the most satisfactory method is the use of artificial exercise in the form of electrical stimulation, because this maintains the metabolism of the muscle and so the size of the fibres.

Physiotherapy can do a great deal to prevent or relieve the trophic changes which tend to occur in the skin, joints, muscles and bones of patients suffering from neurological disorders. Any of these may affect the recovery of voluntary movement.

The object of physical treatment is to stimulate the flow of blood through the area and thus avoid circulatory stasis and increase the nutrition and tissue drainage. The natural stimulus to the circulation is active movement and where possible this method should be used. Thus all the methods in use to gain voluntary movement are also fulfilling this object. Where one segment of a limb is unable to move, active movements of other segments will help to maintain the circulation.

In some cases active movement is impossible and passive measures are necessary. These are particularly important in the cases in which there is vaso-constriction.

Vaso-dilatation will mean a better blood supply and it is produced by heating the tissues. Heat may, therefore, be used directly to the area affected providing, firstly, that there is no sensory loss, and, secondly, that there is not present already a vaso-dilatation due to paralysis of the vaso-constrictor nerves. In either of these cases heat should be applied to the region proximal to the affected area, relying on the fact that there will be a gentler effect on the vessels by the warmed blood entering the area and a lessening of the viscosity of the blood so that it flows more readily in the area of stasis. In addition, there will be a stimulation of the venous and lymphatic flow in the proximal area which will indirectly assist the drainage of the affected area.

Choice between the different sources producing heat depends upon such factors as the condition of cutaneous sensibility and the presence of paralytic vaso-dilatation. If sensation and vaso-motor control are normal inductothermy is a valuable means. Massage is a useful way of stimulating the venous and lymphatic flow and, if there is oedema, it should be carried out with the limb in elevation, but it has to be used with very great care if there is hypertonus or if there is complete atonia, as in the first case it can increase spasticity and in the second it might bruise the flaccid muscle fibres.

Electrical stimulation of the sensory nerve endings and the muscles will help the circulation by stimulating the axon reflex and by increasing metabolism and producing a pumping effect. If oedema is present it is also of value. In the presence of hypertonus this method is better avoided but in cases in which there is hypotonia or atonia the surged faradic or interrupted galvanic currents are useful according to whether the lower motor neurones are conducting impulses or not. If there is no oedema and the first sensory neurones are intact, a sinusoidal bath might be effective, through its stimulating effect on the axon reflex and the warming effect of the hot water.

Sometimes chilblains develop and in this case ultraviolet irradiation or massage with Iodex is often beneficial.

In complete lesions of the spinal cord vaso-motor control is lost, though later some control may be gained through activity of subsidiary spinal centres. For a few weeks following such a lesion there is danger of the development of pressure sores, great care is therefore necessary in nursing and handling the patient and frequent changes of posture are essential. When active movement is permitted constant active changes of posture and vigorous trunk swinging in half suspension will help to re-establish some degree of vaso-motor control.

In treating all patients in whom trophic changes are present, great care of the skin must be taken. It is easily broken down and is slow to heal.

PAIN

Pain will nearly always affect voluntary movement since the patient is not normally willing to move a painful area. Sometimes the pain which limits voluntary movement is arising from the nerve endings in contracted ligaments and peri-articular structures when these structures are stretched on movement. Sometimes the pain is the result of an active inflammatory process in a nerve sheath or in the meninges of the spinal cord. In the first case the only treatment is to continue gentle stretching of the contracted structures. Preceding the stretching by heat often helps to make the movement less painful. In the second case voluntary movements which cause pain should be avoided until the inflammation subsides.

RESTORATION OF INDEPENDENCE

In spite of all that can be done, full recovery may not be possible, but much can be done to give the patient independence in spite of loss of voluntary function. Most important is constant practice in the ward or at home of suitable exercises and occupations. The patient can usually be helped considerably by various 'gadgets'. Thus a tie fitted to a special neck band will enable a man to put on his own tie. A shoe, with a previously fitted elastic lace, and a shoe horn, will save the necessity of someone helping the patient to put his shoe on. Firm bars fitted to the bath-room and bedroom walls will help the patient to stand up, sit down and support himself while washing and dressing.

The patient can also help himself by taking care of his own splints, keeping areas of poor circulation warm, being careful not to damage insensitive areas and doing his own passive movements if these are necessary.

Many different methods have been described in this chapter; some can be used in combination, others may be used alone. Choice of method depends on a variety of factors, the two most important being the age of the patient, and the site and extent of the lesion.

CHAPTER 4

Hemiplegia

REVISED BY TRUDA WAREHAM, M.C.S.P.

HEMIPLEGIA OCCURS commonly in middle age or later life and is then most often the result of a cerebro-vascular accident: cerebral thrombosis or haemorrhage. These are most likely to occur when a degenerative condition of the blood vessels is present and blood pressure is high.

In infancy hemiplegia is either the result of birth injury or occurs in association with one of the specific fevers. In young adults it is likely to be the result of a rupture of the congenital aneurysm or of angioma or of cerebral embolism due either to a small vegetation from a rheumatic or a bacterial endocarditis, or from a clot in any vessel following some surgical procedure. Alternatively, it may result from an intracranial tumour or abscess.

CHANGES

The damage can occur at any level of the corticospinal system, from the cortex to just above the anterior horn cells. The hemiplegia is on the opposite side of the body, unless the lesion occurs below the tract decussation in the hind brain. The variety and severity of the symptoms depend on the site and extent of the lesion, in nearly all cases both the pyramidal and extrapyramidal systems are affected.

SIGNS AND SYMPTOMS

These can be described in three stages:

1. *The onset* is usually sudden, with varying cerebral shock. At one extreme the patient may not lose consciousness, at the other, he may become deeply unconscious for several days.

2. The next stage is characterised by a return of consciousness with flaccidity of arm and leg and, perhaps, face. Tendon reflexes are lost and the plantar response is extensor. Proprioception may be diminished or lost, and balance therefore may be affected.

3. Within a few days or weeks the third stage becomes apparent, with

the gradual onset of spasticity. In untreated severe cases, this may progress to contractures and fixed deformities. Paralysis affecting the dominant side may be accompanied by a wide variety of speech defects.

Incontinence may be present and if the patient remains in bed this may become permanent. The amount of personality change is variable, depending on the amount of brain damage.

The degree of functional activity which will be regained by the patient is, in severe cases, largely dependent on whether skilled physiotherapy is available at once, and whether it can be continued for an adequate period.

PRINCIPLES OF TREATMENT BY PHYSIOTHERAPY

Until consciousness returns treatment, if requested, should consist of a gentle full range passive movement to each joint. If chest complications are present they must be treated by posturing, percussion and suction if necessary.

When consciousness has returned physiotherapy will consist of the following:

1. Explanation and re-assurance to the patient—this is important at every stage.

2. Prevention of stiffness and, later, contractures by means of positioning and by passive and active movements.

3. Training of balance in half lying, sitting on the side of the bed and sitting on a chair; by stabilisation, training the feeling of balance. (The command: 'don't let me push you'.)

4. Training of balance in standing; at first with maximum support, then with decreasing help as recovery occurs.

5. Walking re-training follows the same sequence.

6. Stairs.

7. Mat work—and moving in the bed. Some details of these are given below, but it must be stressed that these do *not* form a simple progression. One does not wait for a patient to be able to balance in standing, before starting to walk, or wait for walking to be free, before starting stairs. Many patients can manage a little of each of these before becoming proficient at the preceding one; in fact, most patients find stairs easier than walking on the flat, and walking usually improves as soon as mat work is started. With a severe stroke caused by cerebral thrombosis and after return to consciousness the following is a rough guide of the programme:

Standing: first or second day.

Walking, sitting down and standing up: first to third day.

Stairs: tenth to fourteenth day.

Mat work: fourteenth to sixteenth day.

By the third week the treatment should, ideally, consist of several short sessions with rest periods so that each part of the programme is covered.

Positioning of the limbs in bed and chair. The possible deformity which in untreated cases might later occur, must be borne in mind and, whenever possible, this must be prevented and the spastic pattern broken up.

In the lower limb the foot tends to become plantar-flexed and inverted, the knee extended, and the hip flexed and adducted. To counter this, the foot should whenever possible be dorsi-flexed, and as soon as possible the patient should sit in a chair, the knee flexed and the foot dorsiflexed. Early ambulation is the most important preventative factor.

In the upper limb, the tendency is for the scapula to become retracted, the shoulder adducted, the elbow flexed, the forearm pronated and the wrist and fingers flexed.

To counter this, two methods are of value: first, inhibitory positioning, the arm being supported on a pillow well in front of the trunk to prevent it and the scapula from falling into extension, second, even more important, full range movements must be given to all joints daily.

Balance in sitting. Sitting on the side of the bed is difficult and patients must be taught to overcorrect, by leaning onto the outstretched good hand. Sitting on a stool or chair is much easier and within a day or two an increasing period should be spent out of bed in a suitable upright high backed chair.

Balance in standing and walking. To accomplish this, the physiotherapist must take up the supporting position. She stands in stride standing facing the patient's paralysed side, one hand in the axilla, the other round the patient's waist—her front knee presses gently on the patient's paralysed leg, so as to lock the knee into extension (Fig. 9a). The patient leans on a tripod or tetrapod held in his good hand. The commands for walking are, 'stick forward', 'good leg forward'. At this command the physiotherapist must give the forward impetus with her own body, and a lift with her hands (9b). Finally at the third command 'bad leg forward', she will assist the weak leg with her foot from behind the patient (Fig. 9c). She then immediately locks it with her forward knee. Such terms as 'good' and 'bad' have to be used, as they cannot understand 'left' and 'right'. If the patient is very big and heavy a more powerful supporting position can be used. The physiotherapist places her shoulder in the patient's axilla, his weak arm over her other shoulder, she places her forward foot well ahead from the patient, and locks his knee with her other knee (Fig. 9d).

Walking is progressed each day by increasing the distance and reducing the amount of support given. At first it is easier to walk with bare feet, later firm walking shoes should be worn.

Balance in standing. This must be practised again and again holding on to the foot of the bed or other stable object. Inversion spasm of the foot can

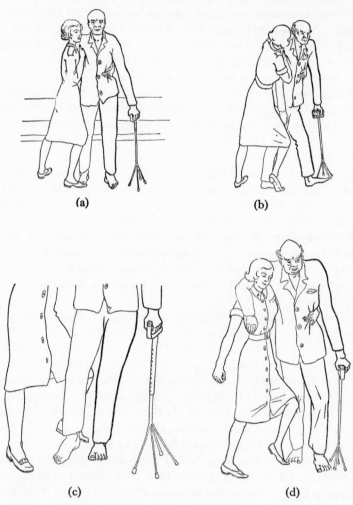

(a)

(b)

(c)

(d)

Fig. 9. Balance in standing and walking.

best be overcome by strengthening the peroneus longus muscle, by making the patient stand and balance on his weak leg trying to get the weight through his big toe.

Mat work is an essential part of the programme. It helps to retrain free hip movements, trunk control, pelvic and scapular control. Patients cannot fall, and so become less anxious and can concentrate on more natural movement.

At the first session it is usually enough to get down to the floor (Fig. 10), move sideways on hand and hip, be helped on to the knees and from there to get back on to a chair (Fig. 11 a and b).

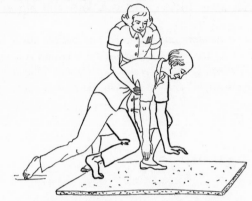

Fig. 10. Getting down to the floor.

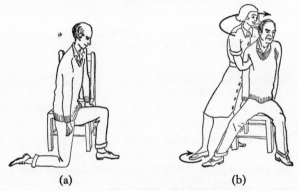

(a)   (b)

Fig. 11. Getting back on to a chair.

Subsequent sessions can teach rolling; first to the weak side, then to the normal side and then how to move up and down in bed using the normal foot and elbow (Fig. 12).

Resisted pelvic and scapular movements are of great value. Crawling, walking on the knees are all gradually introduced. If the patient has painful arthritic joints mat work may have to be omitted.

Stairs. Going up and down stairs is done in the reverse of the usual way. To go up the weak foot is lifted up on to the step, the patient moves his hand up the rail and the physiotherapist gives a helping heave as he steps up. She immediately locks his knee. Even an apparently flail leg will often be tricked into action.

To go down, the hand moves down the rail, the physiotherapist steps down with her own forward leg, and the patient then steps down with his normal leg, thus again tricking the weak knee and hip extensors into paying out.

Knee control in standing and walking. The patient must be taught to appreciate the difference between bracing the knee and relaxing it. This is taught in walk-standing, the affected foot behind. The commands are: 'Hold your knee straight' and 'relax'. On the second command the knee

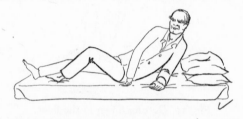

Fig. 12. How to move up and down in bed.
A. Dig the heel in and push.
B. Dig the elbow in and push.
c. Lift the hips and the whole body up off the bed.

is gently flexed. When the patient can balance in standing, this is incorporated in the walking technique. This emphasis on swinging a relaxed, flexed knee forward is important in obtaining a normal gait.

Final stages of walking. Once the hip flexors are working, normal stick and leg gait can be allowed, emphasising full extension of the knee on weight-bearing, and the forward swing with a relaxed knee, the heel striking first. Later resisted walking, forwards, sideways and backwards and all forms of activities can be introduced.

The arm. In the early stages the aim is to maintain the full range of movement. Later positioning and holding in reflex inhibiting postures are practised. These aim at complete relaxation in a position that is totally in opposition to the position of spasm. For example one should aim at holding the upper limb with forward rotation and elevation of the scapula, outward rotation and elevation of the arm, extension of elbow, wrist and fingers, with supination. These holdings should not cause pain. Attempts at active holding should follow.

Active re-education. This is a slow arduous process and is not always successful. A rough guide is as follows. If only minimal voluntary power is present in the shoulder after three months with nothing in the triceps, there is unlikely to be any useful recovery. The patient should be encouraged to accept this fact, and to realise the importance of maintaining a full passive range and so preventing contractures. If after three months there is definite control of scapula, shoulder and triceps, then every effort should be made to continue with re-education as considerable and useful recovery is likely to occur if treatment is given.

Scapular control is gained by scapular movements 'in pattern', and by weight-bearing on the mats or couch in prone, side-lying and on all fours.

Shoulder movements. As in the lower limb isometric contraction usually returns before isotonic, so 'holdings' should follow passive inhibitions. These are followed by eccentric contraction in pattern, and finally isotonic contraction, stressing rotation. As distal recovery occurs it is essential to maintain and increase shoulder control, therefore these exercises must never be omitted, and always form the start of the treatment.

Elbow. Irradiation should be obtained from the shoulder following the same sequence, isometric, eccentric, isotonic, concentric. Only when triceps control is well established, can progression be made to flexion with supination. Weight-bearing on the extended elbow is very useful.

Wrist and hand. Re-education follows the same sequence, all the stress being in extension. A useful inhibiting posture is prone lying with the hand on the sacrum.

Other treatments. Ice can be useful in reducing spasm and is usually better than infra-red irradiation.

With early ambulation a caliper should rarely be needed and then only if the inversion spasm is really severe. If ordered, the best type is an outside iron with a foot lock and a flat rod and socket to the heel, never a toe-spring which tends to increase spasm of the calf.

A night splint is sometimes ordered for the hand in severe cases where there is no recovery; its function is to prevent flexion contractures.

Disseminated Sclerosis. The Parkinsonian Syndrome. Subacute Combined Degeneration of the Cord

DISSEMINATED SCLEROSIS

THIS IS A chronic disease affecting the brain and spinal cord and producing a very wide variety of symptoms. Women are more commonly attacked than men, usually in early adult life.

The cause of the condition is unknown though there is now a theory that disturbance in the circulation to the white matter of the brain and spinal cord, producing transient or permanent ischaemia, may have a bearing on the development of the lesions. An attack sometimes seems to be precipitated by shock, worry or some illness which temporarily confines the patient to bed.

CHANGES

Small lesions may occur anywhere in the white matter of the brain and spinal cord particularly in the optic nerve and optic chiasma, midbrain, pons, cerebellar peduncles and cerebellar tracts and in the lateral columns, and occasionally the posterior columns, of the spinal cord. Less commonly a few may occur in the grey matter.

At the site of the lesion the myelin sheaths disintegrate, there may be a destruction of the axis cylinders and there is a marked increase in the connective tissue. Thus a little patch of scar tissue results. These patches stand out as clearly defined, pinkish-grey areas. At first they are widely scattered and produce only transient symptoms which may completely disappear as undamaged neurones take over, but as the disease progresses and patches of scar tissue fuse more marked and permanent symptoms appear.

Noticeable characteristics of the disease are its tendency to exacerbations and remissions and the varying nature of the symptoms.

SIGNS AND SYMPTOMS

Since the patches of scar tissue may occur almost anywhere in the white matter the onset differs from patient to patient. The optic nerve and optic chiasma are often affected early and blurring of vision may be the first symptom. Tenderness of the eyeballs on pressure and pain will lead to a diagnosis of retro-bulbar neuritis—a diagnosis which in young people is very often a guide to the recognition of early disseminated sclerosis. Paresis of ocular muscles due to lesions in mid-brain or pons may lead to diplopia, ptosis or strabismus, though these are less common early signs. These eye symptoms may last for only a few days, then pass off and no further symptoms appear for some months or even years. The next attack may affect the same area or it may attack other areas and new symptoms and signs may develop such as slight frequency in micturition, paraesthesia, a feeling of heaviness in one leg which tends to drag a little, exaggerated deep reflexes and loss of superficial abdominal reflexes.

When the condition is more advanced and symptoms more stable, the characteristics of the disease will depend upon the region showing most sclerosis. Cases then roughly fall into certain groups, though it is necessary to bear in mind that, though the symptoms of one lesion predominate, other symptoms will be present. For purpose of treatment by physical measures, patients suffering from this disease may be divided into those in whom the lesion is most marked in the cerebellar system and those in whom the incidence is heaviest in the lateral columns of the spinal cord. A few patients will show predominant symptoms arising as a result of lesions in the posterior columns.

Many patients show mental changes and euphoria is the most striking.

In nearly all patients the legs are most affected, the nerve fibres to the legs presenting a longer course to be attacked.

Cerebellar type. Here there are two outstanding features: muscular weakness and hypotonia; and inco-ordination of movement. The hypotonia may be such that the initiation of voluntary movement is difficult. Almost complete loss of power in the legs is not an uncommon feature in advanced cases of this type.

Inco-ordination is the result of hypotonia and lack of postural fixation. A marked side-to-side movement, intention tremor, is seen on movement particularly as the limb nears the object. Overshooting of the mark results from inability on the part of the hypotonic antagonists to slow the movement down. In some patients a movement could be performed if it were not for lack of fixation of some part of the body. Thus walking may be difficult because the pelvis is not stable, taking food to the mouth impaired because of instability of the trunk and head. Nystagmus, oscillation of the eyeballs as the eyes are rotated to one side, is due to inability to co-ordinate the action of the ocular muscles. Dysarthria arises from inability to co-ordinate the lips, larynx and tongue, and is manifested in the form of slurring of speech.

The combination of weakness and lack of fixation produces a staggering gait rather resembling that of a drunken man. This ataxia is at first only noticed when turning, walking round objects or going up and down stairs. Gradually the ataxia increases until the patient cannot walk without aid.

In addition to these signs and symptoms there may also be paraesthesiae, exaggerated reflexes, and extensor plantar response, and some cutaneous sensory impairment. These are due to lesions in other areas of white matter.

The Upper Motor Neurone type. Here increased muscle tone and exaggerated reflexes are the characteristic feature. There is a fairly usual progression of symptoms in these patients. The condition begins with slight increase in tone of the calf muscles, and poverty of dorsiflexion so that the toe is dragged in walking. The legs feel heavy and tire easily. There will be an extensor plantar response and exaggeration of the tendon jerks. Gradually spasticity increases until the total spastic pattern of extension, adduction and medial rotation has developed. Knee and ankle clonus are present and the superficial abdominal reflexes are lost. The patient may complain of numbness and the vibration sense may be diminished.

Later more lesions develop and flexor spasms begin to appear. At first these may be only occasional and slight, but they gradually increase until little stimulus is required to produce them. Eventually the total spastic pattern may change to flexion, abduction and lateral rotation. Adaptive shortening of muscle and fascia occurs, tendon organs are irritated by the contracted state of tendons, and the legs become fixed in flexion, abduction and lateral rotation.

The trunk is also often involved and unsupported sitting may be difficult. Some degree of cerebellar ataxia may also be present.

Patients with advanced upper motor neurone lesions usually suffer more than those of the cerebellar type because flexion spasms are painful, and sores easily develop on prominent bony points which, due to the deformity, are abnormally exposed to friction and pressure. Bladder troubles are also often present.

Sensory ataxia. In some patients the posterior columns of the cord are most affected. Kinaesthetic sense is then impaired. The patient, unaware of the position of his joints, is unable to perform co-ordinated movement. Walking becomes ataxic and if cutaneous sensation in the soles of the feet is impaired the gait will closely resemble that of the diabetic patient.

There will also almost always be some evidence of involvement of the lateral columns and cerebellar peduncles.

PRINCIPLES OF PHYSIOTHERAPY TREATMENT

The objects and means of treatment vary according to the outstanding symptoms and their severity. Other factors such as impairment of vision and sensation have to be taken into account. In more advanced cases it is important to know whether it is actually possible to keep the patient ambulant or whether the patient must be equipped with a wheel-chair. As in all chronic diseases the final aim is to get the patient as independent as is possible. The first step, therefore, is a careful examination on the lines indicated in Chapter 2.

This should enlighten the physiotherapist as to the nature and severity of the main symptoms, the area of the body affected, the state of the patient's vision and the degree of independence in the activities of daily living.

The Cerebellar and Sensory types. The main objects of physiotherapy are to strengthen the muscles, gain good postural fixation and improve co-ordination. Proprioceptive facilitation techniques should be used to gain the greatest number of afferent impulses so that all motor areas including cerebellum, cortex and subcortical areas are stimulated as strongly as possible. Maximal resistance, approximation or traction, stretch, touch, sight and hearing should all be used.

In giving the stretch stimulus it should be remembered that movements are usually diagonal and spiral in character. Before starting the passive or active movements all components should be fully stretched. This will automatically lead to the performance of a mass movement pattern.

Constant repetition is very important and the patient's attention must be closely held because in these ways it is hoped that alternative pathways will be established and dormant neurones activated.

These methods may be applied to the exercises designed by Dr. Frankel so that modified Frankel exercises are used.

Mass movement patterns may be adapted to gain overflow from stronger to weaker muscle groups. By exercising the stronger components of a movement the weaker components will be facilitated. To improve power the technique of repeated contraction may be used. These may be done at first without a 'hold' at any point in the range and later, as the patient's ability improves, with a 'hold' at the strongest point in the range of movement where the maximum number of motor units can be activated.

N

Slow reversals should be substituted as power improves. This is because the patient is now able to concentrate on two patterns of movement. As the patient improves progression is made to rhythmic stabilisations.

If patients have problems with speech the same principles will be applied to the muscles of respiration, face, larynx and tongue.

Stimulus to the contraction of muscle groups can be obtained by stroking the skin over the groups with crushed ice and swallowing can be stimulated by the use of spicy drinks, such as Bovril or soups.

Mat work is an essential part of the treatment since it introduces daily activities and on either a high mat or on a mat on the floor the patient has confidence and is not afraid of falling.

Exercises should begin at the stage the particular patient has reached. One patient may need to start with rolling from prone to supine, another may be capable of rolling but not of sitting up from lying. A brief idea of the stages of progression would be as follows: prone lying gaining head control; prone lying with forearm support, and rolling into the supine position; rolling from supine to prone (more difficult because of the extra head control needed); prone lying with forearm support changing to side sitting; prone lying with forearm support changing to prone kneeling; high kneeling in front of a stool or chair with hands on chair; half kneeling; standing; walking; walking sideways and backwards; walking on slopes and upstairs; walking on rough surfaces and learning to fall and to get up.

Some patients, particularly the elderly, are unable to take prone kneeling or kneeling. These patients will be helped from side sitting to sitting. In the sitting position they are taught to lean forward and place the hands on a stool in front and to the side and to stand up from this position.

In each position the patient has to learn to balance and rhythmic stabilisation will help here. She also has to learn to move forwards, backwards and sideways and directional resistance is valuable to assist this.

Other functional activities such as sitting on the edge of the bed, dressing, changing from bed to chair, going to the toilet and bath, getting into and out of a chair must be practised.

One particular point to bear in mind is the special importance of gaining stability of the head and trunk. If the head is unsteady it is almost impossible to co-ordinate movements of the limbs. A great deal of attention should therefore be paid to rhythmic stabilisation using approximation. Many of these patients seem to respond better to 'holdings' than to actual movement.

The Spastic type. For these patients voluntary movement is difficult because of the spasticity. The first object is therefore to try to reduce spasticity by whatever means seems to be most effective for each patient.

Rhythmical passive movements are often very valuable. Here rotation of the trunk is particularly important. It facilitates the righting reflexes which in their turn exert an inhibitory influence over tonic reflexes, which, in spasticity, may have been released from control.

Ice towels applied from origin to insertion of spastic muscle groups will often markedly reduce the tone.

Facilitation techniques using repeated contractions and slow reversals can be most effective but they require great skill because if not carefully performed spasticity may actually be increased. Some physiotherapists prefer therefore to use other methods.

Choice of the position from which movements are performed is vital if spasticity is to be reduced and movement encouraged. Recalling that for the legs the total patterns of spasticity are extension, adduction and medial rotation, and flexion, abduction and lateral rotation, the position from which movement is tried must be such that one or more of the components of these patterns are altered. Side sitting is an excellent example of this since in left side sitting the left leg is in flexion, *adduction* and lateral rotation, and the right leg is in relative extension, *abduction* and medial rotation.

When spasticity has been reduced the patient is encouraged to try simple movements in the reflex inhibiting patterns such as in side lying and side sitting. It is often found that these are better done without resistance. This depends on the particular patient; in some, resistance increases spasticity, in others directional resistance is helpful.

Mat work and functional activities are essential as for the cerebellar type of disseminated sclerosis.

Some advanced cases with flexion contractures will need training in the use of a wheel chair and this can, if it does not increase spasticity, be carried out against directional resistance. These patients will also require particular attention to the trunk and arm muscles.

In all types of disseminated sclerosis the emphasis lies on assessing the patient, finding out what she cannot do and working to get her to master the difficulty. Hard and constant work are the keynotes. Probably it is wiser not to work the patient to the point of real fatigue. If signs of fatigue begin to appear the treatment should be reassessed.

There is a school of thought which, believing that interference with circulation is the possible cause of the lesions, uses vigorous exercises repeated a definite number of times several periods daily as the method of choice in treating these patients.

Whatever method is chosen the ideal is to start treatment as early as possible before the disease has started to progress.

THE PARKINSONIAN SYNDROME

This is a disturbance of motor function named after Dr. James Parkinson who first described it. The syndrome is characterised by tremor, rigidity, and the gradual slowing and weakening of voluntary and emotional movements.

There is degeneration of the cells of the basal ganglia particularly in the corpus striatum and substantia nigra. This degeneration may follow chronic encephalitis lethargica, or may be due to cerebral arteriosclerosis, or it may be a primary degeneration of unknown origin.

The same characteristics are present whatever the cause, but other symptoms will also be present if the disease is associated with cerebral vascular disorders.

SIGNS AND SYMPTOMS

These usually begin to appear between the ages of 50 and 60 in paralysis agitans, earlier if the syndrome follows encephalitis and rather later in cerebral arteriosclerosis, though in the latter case it progresses more rapidly.

Tremor. In paralysis agitans this is usually the first symptom, but if the condition follows encephalitis it often appears later, some time after rigidity has developed. Tremor consists of a rhythmical alternating contraction of opposing muscle groups at the rate of about four to eight per second. It often ceases during voluntary movement of the limb, is absent during sleep but appears when the limb is not being used, especially if it is unsupported. Usually it commences in the fingers and thumb of one hand resulting in a 'pill-rolling' movement. It then spreads to a flexion and extension of the wrist and to pronation and supination of the forearm. In many cases the leg of the same side is next affected, flexion and extension of the ankle being most marked. Tremor may then spread to the opposite arm and leg. The head is also involved, either a rotatory movement or flexion and extension occurring. The jaw may rhythmically open and close and the tongue protrude and retract.

Tremor is not usually marked in Parkinsonism due to cerebral arteriosclerosis, though a senile tremor may be present. This differs in that it is quicker and finer, not usually present at rest, but present on voluntary movement. It is more frequent in the muscles of the head and is not associated with rigidity.

Rigidity. This is an increase in tone which is equal in all muscle groups. It is maintained throughout the whole range of movement of a joint, though full range can nearly always be obtained passively unless contractures have developed. If tremor is also present the muscles yield in a series of jerks as passive movements are performed. The term 'cog-wheel' rigidity is used in this case. If tremor is not present the rigidity is smooth and this is known as the 'lead-pipe' rigidity.

Disorders of movement. Difficulty in initiating movement, weakness and slowness of voluntary movement are present whatever the cause. They are particularly noticeable in the small muscles and fine movements. Speech becomes slurred and monotonous, mastication slow and difficult. Movements of the fingers are clumsy and writing, tying laces, doing up buttons, dressing, using a knife or razor all become increasingly difficult.

Some associated and synergic movements are lost, swinging of the arms in walking is reduced and extension of the wrist when the fingers are flexed is diminished, interfering with grip.

Weakness of emotional movements together with rigidity give the patient a peculiar masklike expression known as the Parkinsonian mask. Blinking is infrequent, the eyes stare, the mouth is slightly open, the face fails to light up in conversation. Smiling is slow to develop and slow to disappear.

Weakness and rigidity are responsible for alterations in posture and gait. The head is usually bent, the trunk flexed, the arms adducted and flexed, forearms pronated, fingers bent at the metacarpo-phalangeal joints and straight at the interphalangeal joints, the thumb lying against the palmar surface of the index finger. Knees and hips are slightly flexed. In this position the centre of gravity tends to fall towards the front of the base and balance is easily upset. The patient takes short, shuffling steps and cannot stop quickly if pushed forward or backward. Often he can carry out small range rapid movements more easily than slow large movements so that it is easier to walk quickly than slowly.

Reflexes. These are difficult to elicit and are reduced in amplitude due to rigidity but the plantar response is usually a normal flexor one.

Autonomic symptoms. Excessive salivation and sweating, flushing of the skin and uncomfortable sensations of heat often give rise to considerable discomfort.

The condition is progressive and eventually activity becomes increasingly limited until the patient is almost completely immobile. The mental state usually remains normal except when the condition is due to cerebral vascular disorders when there is often mental deterioration.

PRINCIPLES OF TREATMENT BY PHYSIOTHERAPY

Though the Parkinsonian syndrome is incurable, considerable relief of discomfort and improvement of function can be obtained. One important object of physiotherapy is to make the patient 'safe'. Because of rigidity his great difficulty is in balance. Thus it is important to train him to make the necessary adjustments to keep the centre of gravity over the base. Other objects are: to gain larger, freer movements; to improve chest expansion and ability to cough; to maintain full range of joint movements; to strengthen muscle power and maintain independence.

While different methods are available one method economical of time is the use of mass movement patterns with proprioceptive neuro-muscular facilitation. Since initiation of voluntary movement is a problem the rhythm technique is used and since rigidity makes movement difficult ice therapy may be used to relax the muscles. Ice towels are applied to muscle groups from origin to insertion and changed frequently. This may be done while other areas are being treated. The rhythm technique is used for all patterns of movement all over the body, including movements of the jaw, tongue, and swallowing. A pattern is chosen and the patient asked to let the physiotherapist do the movement. The movement is performed passively in as full a range as possible. As the patient begins to 'let go' he is asked to try to assist, gradually resistance is added and eventually the patient does the movement freely. The opposite pattern is then carried out in the same way. This method achieves a larger, easier movement. The same technique is applied to mat work. This work begins at whatever stage the patient has reached in the normal development sequence. Some patients may need to be taught rolling, this is again done first passively, then as an assisted active movement, then resisted, then freely. This is progressed through the various stages to sitting and standing. In each position balance is gained by the use of approximation of joint surfaces, so stimulating the kinaesthetic sense and therefore gaining an extensor response. The patient is also taught to move in this position.

Re-education of walking is started at the same time. The essential point is to exaggerate all movements. The patient is taught to get up from sitting, first learning to lean forward. This is done with the same rhythm technique. He is then taught to stand up in the same way. Next, between parallel bars, he is taught high stepping on the spot using the same technique. When the legs are working well, arm swinging is taught, then the arms and legs are combined. Walking in a large circle follows, the physiotherapist giving directional guidance on pelvis, shoulders or arms where necessary. The next progression is walking in a figure of eight in which some turning movement is involved. The patient is then taught to stop to command and to start again without a shuffling gait. He then tries walking straight forward, stopping and turning to command.

Throughout, the physiotherapist does the same movements with the patient and encourages exaggerated movements. By doing exaggerated movement it is hoped that the patient will gradually be able to use normal range instead of the small movements he has been doing.

The use of the rhythm technique in *rotation* of the trunk and limbs seems to be particularly helpful. It frees movement and can then be followed by stimulation of semi-automatic responses. For example, with the patient sitting and a stool in front and to one side, passive trunk rotation is started. Gradually the patient joins in and as soon as he is doing the movement on his own freely he is encouraged as he rotates to lean forward and let his hands rest on the stool. Then the suggestion 'now let's stand' is given and from this position he is gently pushed into standing and encouraged to walk forwards. Often it is now found that walking is much freer and he can continue turning and walking back to the chair and sitting down.

Home exercises are essential. They must be simple and a relative can be taught to help. Thus, for example, he can practise the mat exercises and high stepping. Activities which the patient normally enjoys should be encouraged; swinging a golf club, playing ball games with children, taking the dog for a walk, are more beneficial than set exercises if the patient enjoys them.

The patient should be advised not to rest on his back because this increases rigidity and to push rather than pull himself up for the same reason.

SURGICAL TREATMENT

A great progression in the treatment of the Parkinsonian syndrome is stereotaxic surgery under local anaesthesia. Coagulation of small areas of the globus pallidus and anterolateral nucleus of the thalamus is carried out through a burr hole in the skull. This is usually successful in reducing tremor and rigidity in the limbs.

The patient gets up and walks on the second post-operative day and he can join a class of other patients on the third day. The lines of treatment follow those for the conservative method but since rigidity and tremor are reduced or relieved progression is much more rapid.

In both conservative and surgical treatments attention must be paid to training the patient in dressing, feeding and toilet activities. He may be helped if necessary by the use of gadgets, the substitution of zips for buttons, thicker handles on knife, fork, spoon, brush and comb, and elastic shoe-laces. These patients tire very easily and everything should be made as easy as possible. Encouragement is needed to keep the patient going out and meeting other people because he is conscious of his changed appearance and speech problems.

SUBACUTE COMBINED DEGENERATION OF THE CORD

This is a progressive degenerative disease associated with a deficiency of Vitamin B_{12}, so that it is sometimes known as Vitamin B_{12} neuropathy. The majority of patients suffer also from pernicious anaemia but this may be slight and is sometimes absent. The onset is usually about the age of 50 and both sexes are equally affected.

CHANGES

The changes are those of demyelination of the nerve fibres and, in severe cases, destruction of the axons. These changes appear first in the lower cervical and upper thoracic regions of the spinal cord and affect the posterior and lateral columns. Similar changes occur in the peripheral nerves and sometimes in the white matter of the brain.

SIGNS AND SYMPTOMS

The onset is usually gradual, the patient first complaining of tingling, numbness and coldness in the toes. The paraesthesia spreads upwards to the trunk and later occurs in the arms, starting in the tips of the fingers. At the same time kinaesthetic sensation is diminished and there is loss of cutaneous sensibility to light touch, heat and cold, and pinprick. This is noticed first in the feet, later in the hands giving rise to the 'stocking and glove' distribution of sensory loss. Numbness of the fingers leads to clumsiness in the fine movements of the hands.

Gradually ataxia, weakness and spasticity develop, the predominant symptom depending on which part of the spinal cord is most affected. If the posterior column is involved, sensory loss and sensory ataxia will be most noticeable and Rhomberg's sign will be present. If the lateral column is most affected, spasticity with extensor plantar response will be the outstanding feature. Due to the degeneration of peripheral nerves there will be muscle weakness and atrophy, loss of ankle and knee jerks and disturbance of sensation. In many patients sphincter disturbances also occur. Symptoms of pernicious anaemia are present in some cases. There are gastro-intestinal disturbances, a yellowish tint of the skin with a bright malar flush, swelling of the feet and ankles, breathlessness on exertion and pallor of the lips and mucous membranes.

PROGNOSIS

The disease can be arrested by the administration of Vitamin B_{12} but whether the symptoms are relieved depends on the degree of degeneration reached before treatment is started. Peripheral nerves can regenerate and weakness and atrophy will then disappear, but severe sensory ataxia and spasticity would persist.

PHYSIOTHERAPY TREATMENT

This depends on the predominant symptoms and a careful examination must be carried out (see Chap. 2). It will follow the principles discussed for muscle weakness, sensory ataxia or spasticity (see Chap. 3), but in addition it must include training of sensation and instructions to the patient about care of the hands and feet if there is cutaneous sensory loss.

CHAPTER 6

Cerebral Palsy

BY DOREEN ALLEN, S.R.N., M.C.S.P., Dip.T.P.

CEREBRAL PALSY IS THE TERM given to those disorders of the motor system caused by damage or malfunction of the central nervous system in the infant or young child. Muscle spasticity is the commonest result of such damage and the patients are often referred to as 'spastics'.

AETIOLOGY Cerebral palsy may be congenital or acquired.

1. Agenesis. A defective development of neurones in the brain.

2. Trauma. Intracranial injury of neurones, especially due to oxygen deprivation.

3. Kernicterus.

4. Infection.

5. Vascular accident.

The lesion may occur during:

Prenatal life—Antepartum haemorrhage, severe toxaemia or a prolonged labour may interfere with the placental circulation.

Delivery—A precipitate birth resulting in shock and difficulty in establishing respiration, especially in premature infants.

Neonatal period—Severe jaundice and anaemia usually associated with either Rhesus incompatibility or prematurity.

Cerebral palsy may be acquired from birth up to three-years-old—resulting from meningitis, encephalitis or following measles, whooping cough, immunization or vaccination.

CLINICAL FEATURES

In view of the many possible causes it is understandable that the damage may be severe with devastating results. Every kind of injury to the nervous system may be seen in different patients. On the other hand the damage may be minimal, so that the child is no more than clumsy or slow, or may stutter. He can become frustrated because hand skills are spoilt by excessive activity of the flexor muscles, so that he grips his pen too tightly, and in addition may not be able properly to dissociate his finger movements.

Early signs and symptoms

1. The baby is abnormally still and quiet, or overactive with an irritable cry.
2. Failure to suck properly.
3. Infant motor skills ('milestones') are not developing properly.

Later

4. *Abnormal reflex activity*

(*a*) Abnormal patterns of posture and movement are seen.

(*b*) Muscle may be hypertonic (spastic), hypotonic (flaccid) or variable—tone may appear normal at rest, becoming hypertonic on effort, collapsing into hypotonia.

(*c*) Brisk reflexes, indicating damage to the inhibitory centres and pathways of the central nervous system.

5. Muscle weakness may be present.
6. Varying degrees of defective proprioceptive and cutaneous sensation, especially in the hemiplegic patient.
7. Special senses may be involved—there may be aphasia, deafness, especially high tone deafness, squints and visual defects.
8. Mentally these patients may be in any part of the normal range or defective. The majority are probably of a low average. It is important when assessing intelligence to consider each feature of the child's handicap, and especially his lack of sensory experience due to motor difficulties. Because of clenched hands and the inability to bring the arms together, he may never have been able to play with his hands and toes, touch his body, suck his fingers and so learn the body image. There may be a defective response to pressure from hands and feet which have never received the normal stimulus of weight-bearing.
9. Epilepsy. Fits may occur from birth, or develop subsequently.
10. Atrophy of limb(s), accompanied by poor circulation. This defective growth tends to become more marked as the child gets older. It is not necessarily associated with abnormal muscle tone or lack of use, and it is by no means constantly present.

DISTRIBUTION OF NEURO-MUSCULAR INVOLVEMENT

Diplegia—the whole child is affected, the lower limbs more severely than the upper.

Bilateral Hemiplegia—the whole child is affected, the upper limbs more severely than the lower.

Triplegia—one limb, usually an arm, is normal.

Paraplegia—the lower half of the body is affected.

Hemiplegia—one side of the body is affected (*see* Plate XII).

Monoplegia—one limb is involved.

Type of neuro-muscular involvement

Spastic

Athetoid—athetosis is characterised by involuntary movements. Muscle tone fluctuates (variable). The maintenance of postures, control throughout a range of movement and the response to gravity, i.e. the ability to bear weight, are all impaired. Static muscle work, eccentric-muscle work, and co-contraction are difficult. The patient is inco-ordinated, but has a good repertoire of movement.

Variable rigidity—simulates athetosis, but without involuntary movements.

Ataxic—hypotonia—there is difficulty in maintaining postures. Movements may be strong, but jerky and inco-ordinated.

In any one patient there may be a combination of these signs, of which spasticity associated with athetosis is the commonest. All types show abnormal reflex activity, and the control of these pathological reflexes by using reflex inhibiting postures is the basic principle of treatment.

EXAMINATION OF PATIENT

Preparation of Patient. Infants and little children are often distressed if undressed, therefore this should be delayed.

Every treatment should be an examination and assessment of the condition: abnormal attitudes and abnormal movements should be noted throughout the examination. For instance, the head may be always turned or rotated to one side; there may be an increase of extensor spasticity as the patient is turned on to his back (the tonic labyrinthine reflex); the apparently floppy head which the infant is unable to lift may be due to extensor spasticity of the neck; the toes that look normal may become spastic on effort, e.g. when the patient uses his hands, or perhaps when he talks; the hemiplegic patient may always turn round towards his sound side.

A. Testing reflex activity

1. *Passive movements* are given to every part of the body, and careful observation is made of muscle tone and the range of movement. To gain a full range of movement must be a primary aim of treatment. The muscles

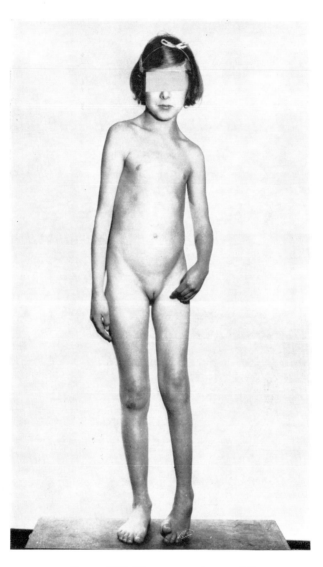

PLATE XII. HEMIPLEGIA (*see p.* 186)
Showing atrophy of the left side

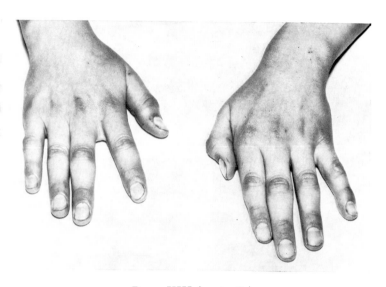

PLATE XIII (*see p.* 187)

TESTING REFLEX ACTIVITY IN THE HANDS

(a) Showing non-abduction of thumb and index finger

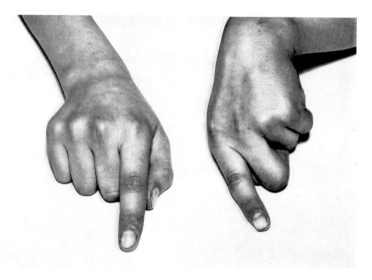

(b) Showing non-extension of index finger

which tend to be most spastic, and if neglected lead to stiff joints as the child gets older, are the plantar flexors, hamstring muscles, adductors of the wrist and pronators of the forearm.

2. *Passive postures* (*see* Fig. 13) such as arms crossed on chest, tailor sitting, standing.

The Bobath grading of postures and movements is a useful method of assessment

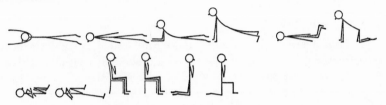

Fig. 13. Postures in testing reflex activities.

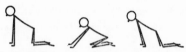

Fig. 14. Movements in testing reflex activities.

Can he be placed in position? No = 0; Yes = 1.
Can he maintain the position, though abnormal = 2.

3. (*a*) *Active Postures*, *see* Figs. 13 and 14.
Can he take the position, though abnormal = 3.
Can he take the position, though slightly abnormal = 4
$$\text{normal} = 5$$
(*b*) Active movements (chart 0, 3, 4, or 5) such as rolling, crawling.

Try to analyse which reflexes are spoiling postures and movements, e.g. sitting may be prevented or spoilt by the excessive activity of either the flexor or extensor groups, and/or by the asymmetric tonic neck reflex where turning the head to the right, the whole of the right side may tend to extend whilst the whole of the left side tends to flex, upsetting sitting balance.

4. *Hands*—test the following abilities:
(*a*) Bimanual use of hands.
(*b*) Dissociation of fingers—flexion/extension. Dissociation of fingers—abduction/adduction. Isolated movements of thumb, of each individual finger.
(*c*) Strength of pressure of each finger and thumb.
(*d*) Use of distal phalanges (*see* Plate XIII A and B).

B. Test muscle power by resisting voluntary movement. There may be damage on the excitory side of the central nervous system to give muscle weakness. When spasticity has been reduced power may be normal, or muscle weakness may then be apparent.

C. Report from parents and patient concerning all activities, play, social life, specific problems, progress or regression, home treatment and appliances.

D. Shoes and Boots

(*a*) *Type*. Spastic feet are often most comfortable in light shoes or sandals, though sometimes in soft supporting shoes or boots. They must fit well. Some patients have one foot smaller than the other, and each shoe requires to be of a different size. If the shoes tend to come off, high lacing, a strap over the foot or round the ankle may be required.

(*b*) Observe always where and how shoes are worn out. Some children are very hard on their shoes. In these cases it may be possible to concentrate treatment on the feet applying an all-round plaster of Paris splint followed by a Swedish splint.

E. Testing of functional activities, adaptation of clothing and other aids and appliances should be discussed with the occupational therapist.

AIMS OF TREATMENT

1. To suppress abnormal reflex activity (or abnormal reflexes and spasticity) by developing the inhibitory function of the nervous system, and thus to improve the pattern of posture and movement of the patient.

2. To stimulate and train the sensory nervous system in proprioception, exteroception and the body image.

3. To gain a full range of movement in every joint.

4. To strengthen muscles if they are weak after spasticity has been reduced.

5. To increase muscle tone and postural control in ataxia and athetosis.

6. To train perception such as spatial appreciation and recognition of shapes.

TREATMENT

The normal maturation of the nervous system during infancy and early childhood consists to a large extent of the development and dominance of higher centres in the brain. Inhibitory mechanisms are an important function of these centres and the motor development of the child may be regarded as the gradual suppression of reflex patterns which were normal at an earlier age. For example, the asymmetric tonic neck reflex of extension of the limb towards which the neck is turned with flexion of the limb on the other side of the body disappears with inhibition during normal development, but may persist in children or re-appear if brain damage occurs at any later date.

The normal inhibitory pathways are defective in cerebral palsy and alternative mechanisms must be trained. The infant is not often paralysed. The ability to hold postures and perform movements is spoilt by abnormal muscle tone and abnormal reflexes. He is limited in what he can do because with every effort his nervous energy passes down wrong pathways, i.e. extensor or flexor reflex patterns, etc. The activities he achieves will be of an abnormal pattern.

The student should study the normal infant because the treatment consists of enabling the infant with cerebral palsy to develop his milestones.

TO TRAIN THE INHIBITORY COMPONENTS OF THE CENTRAL NERVOUS SYSTEM

1. *Reflex Inhibiting Postures*

The patient is placed in the different fundamental starting positions, and any abnormality corrected. It is important to control the whole patient as far as possible. Full range of movement should be obtained and this may be assisted by passive shakings, and the hold relax and the contract relax techniques. The physiotherapist gradually lightens her control as the patient learns to maintain the positions.

Movement in the reflex inhibiting postures is introduced as soon as possible, both passive and active movements commencing in small ranges but in every part of the range of movement. For instance, kneeling, sitting back on the heels and up again and on the floor to either side. Rotation is an important component to exercise. Every variety of posture and movement should be included, for instance, the three components of the neuromuscular facilitation technique, e.g. flexion adduction lateral rotation and extension abduction medial rotation patterns of the leg as well as the straight patterns; the tailor sitting, pulling over on to hands and knees of the infant and all the symmetrical and asymmetrical positions and movements. Limited progress of the patient over the months and years can be due to the fact that the physiotherapist is limited in the variety of postures and movements she uses in treatment.

In cerebral palsy it is more often the supporting part of the body that spoils function rather than the moving part, e.g. the patient cannot use the arms because the sitting position is insecure; may not be able to walk because he cannot stand (hypotonic patient); cannot get up from the prone position because he is unable to support weight on the arms. The aim in treatment should be to improve sitting, standing, weight-bearing on arms. Consolidation of starting positions are best obtained when the patient is distracted, standing, playing with a ball, or with toys on a table that is exactly the right height. During this time the physiotherapist maintains a correct base, e.g. heels down, legs abducted and laterally rotated. She also varies the base in size and in direction. Again, she assesses throughout treatment whether it is possible to decrease her control, without wrong patterns asserting themselves.

Transference of weight is another factor to be included, e.g. the child in a good squatting position; if the physiotherapist transfers the weight to one side, she may enable it to step sideways; or, kneeling, if the weight is passively transferred to one side and controlled, the child may be able to take the half-kneeling position with the other leg.

In treatment the cerebral palsy patient should look normal, because he is being controlled, though this is not always possible with older patients and those severely injured. He must also look active. Treatment should be given in front of mirrors.

As early as possible, the normal righting reflexes should be elicited. For instance, the body righting reflex whereby the body turns segmentally the head, the shoulder girdle on the head and the pelvis on the shoulder girdle. Or the leg and pelvis may be turned first. Thus the normal infant turns from the supine position on to his side. The cerebral palsy child may be prevented by extensor spasticity. He should be passively manoeuvred, at one of these parts of the body, rocking him over on to his side. In a similar way infants may be got on to their hands and knees, to kneel, to stand, to crawl, by passive manoeuvring of their head positions.

Very important are the normal protective reflexes. For instance with the patient in the kneeling position, he is gently pushed off balance forwards, and to either side. Normally the arms extend to take the weight of the body to save falling on the head.

Balance reactions should also be trained in all starting positions. Normally, muscles adjust the body if it is falling outside its base of support. Because of abnormal reflexes and abnormal muscle tone the cerebral palsied patient may be unable to move to regain his balance, even if the base is large as in sitting. Moving the body outside the base whilst helping and encouraging the patient segmentally to recover his balance, must be practised in treatment. It may be done voluntarily, asking the patient to recover his balance; or reflexly, positioning him off balance to stimulate him to recover his balance automatically. Another method is gently, but unexpectedly to push the patient in all directions.

2. *Stimulation of the sensory nervous system*

Proprioception. It is by compression of joints, or traction and the stretching of muscles, and the giving of maximum resistance that contraction can be stimulated either reflexly or voluntarily.

Exteroception. It is by placing the hand over the skin in the direction of the movement that gives the patient the right feel of the movement. The use of the voice is important. Facilitation is used throughout treatment in the reflex inhibiting postures in order to assist normal reflex movement, voluntary movement and the maintenance of postures.

Body image. Parents can be shown how to enable the infant to feel his body, put his fingers in his mouth and gradually to become aware of the relative position of various parts of the body.

3. *Techniques for increasing range of movement*

(*a*) All-round plaster of Paris splint. The object is to hold spastic muscles continuously in the lengthened position and so tire out constant muscle over-activity.

All-round plaster splinting should be done when the child is young, for two main reasons:

(i) The sooner range is gained, and weight-bearing is on a flat foot, the better.

(ii) Children under ten years do not seem to mind splints.

(*b*) Icing—Indicated especially for spastic hamstrings and calf muscles. Use cloths wrung out in flaked ice, or apply bag containing crushed ice. The duration of treatment should be progressively increased from five to twenty minutes.

(*c*) Surgery may be indicated when abnormal reflex activity has been sufficiently reduced, especially if there are contractures in the soft tissues.

4. *To strengthen weak muscles*

Weak muscles can only be strengthened by voluntary action against maximal resistance, and for this both static and active muscle work is required. They should be worked specially in their inner range, using repeated contractions and slow reversal techniques. Train in functional mass patterns of movements and in localised muscle work. Inhibit abnormal reflex patterns throughout treatment. Associated reactions may be disregarded, they are associated with effort. As the muscles strengthen, associated reactions decrease.

o

5. *To increase tone*

Patients with hypotonus may be able to perform strong concentric muscle work, but have difficulty in maintaining postures. The selected starting position must be corrected and reflex abnormality inhibited.

The techniques used are:

(*a*) Heavy tapping and heavy pressure over joints in the endeavour to gain co-contraction of muscles. (Simultaneous contraction of agonists and antagonists.)

(*b*) Rhythmic stabilisation—in all postures, and in every part of the range of movement.

SPLINTAGE

1. *To gain range*

(*a*) All-round plaster of Paris splints are used to tire out hypertonus. They are applicable to the ankle and foot, very occasionally to the wrist and hands (*see* Plate XIV (A)).

(*b*) Abduction leg plasters with foot pieces. They are best made in plaster, as after a few weeks a new splint will be required with an increased range of abduction. The patient should wear the splint for a few hours a day, and be activated in it. Activity increases the spasticity of the leg which the splint inhibits. It is a definite treatment, not to be worn passively. At the right stage of treatment it is valuable for some months (*see* Plate XIV (B)).

2. *To inhibit abnormal reflex patterns* and thereby improve function.

The joints must be sufficiently mobile before the splint is applied.

(*a*) Lively foot-raising below-knee brace (Swedish type).

(*b*) Polythene hand splint (*see* Plate XV (A) and (B)).

(*c*) Collars. The head position has a strong reflex influence over the rest of the body.

HOME TREATMENT

The whole family should be encouraged to help.

1. *General approach*

The physiotherapist should examine the patient with the parents. She must show the parents the most corrective way of carrying the child, its best position in bed, best sitting position, etc. She must explain the importance of a variety of positions, that certain milestones develop from the prone position, etc. and that the child must be encouraged to move, to roll, etc.

The arrangement of household equipment should be checked, for

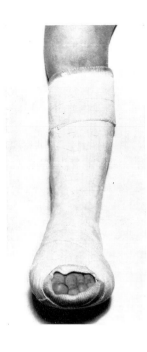

PLATE XIV (*see p.* 192)
(a) Plaster of Paris splint for foot and ankle

(b) Abduction leg plasters with foot pieces

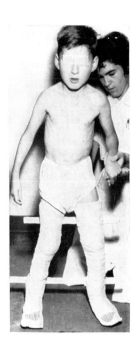

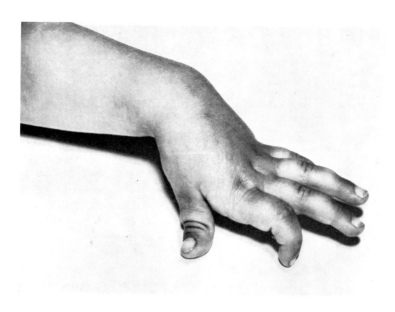

PLATE XV. HANDSPLINTING IN CEREBRAL PALSY (*see p.* 192)
(a) Showing abnormal reflex pattern

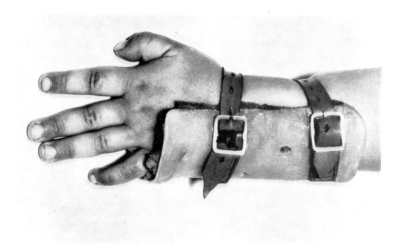

(b) Splint inhibiting abnormal reflex pattern

instance the television should be the right height, so that the child, without getting annoyed, must lift its head to watch.

2. *Sensation and perception*

The child should be encouraged to feel objects of different sizes, shapes, textures and weight; to turn switches and taps on and off, learning to relate the switch going down with the light coming on, the winding of the clock with it beginning to tick, etc.

3. *Specific treatment*

The reflex inhibiting postures and controlled movements must be carefully chosen so that they are not too difficult for the parents to do properly, yet difficult enough to be a valuable training for the nervous system.

4. *Lifting*

Parents should be taught the proper way to lift as the child gets older.

ASSESSMENT OF PROGRESS

1. Postures and movements should be recorded regularly by a definite system, e.g. the Bobath grading.

2. Note all improvements in treatment, e.g. abnormal reflexes are less constant or appear more slowly.

3. Note all improvements in functional activities, e.g. parents not being disturbed at night because child is able to turn; able to carry a tray; shoes not being so worn; child not falling so frequently.

It is interesting for the parents or the older child to keep a diary of progress.

OCCUPATIONAL THERAPY

1. Hand activities and the training of sensation and perception should be given in easy reflex inhibiting postures, and in the standing or abduction plasters for the children that have them.

2. In certain patients the use of the hands does not improve simultaneously with the decrease of abnormal reflex activity, especially with hemiplegic patients with some sensory defect. They require bimanual training.

3. From time to time it is important to have a thorough assessment of functional activities.

SPEECH THERAPY

Sucking, chewing, dribbling, speech difficulties and abnormal respiration, are all treated by the speech therapist in co-operation with the physiotherapist. The abnormal jaw and tongue movements are part of the total abnormal reflex pattern. The speech therapist will probably give treatment in the appropriate reflex inhibiting posture, e.g. one that controls the extension of the head, retraction of the shoulder girdle, etc.

Diaphragmatic breathing can usually be stimulated by quick icing, i.e. using an ice cube stroke two or three times on either side of the umbilicus.

Both occupational and speech therapists should use easy reflex inhibiting postures so that they can quickly proceed to their specialised work. The physiotherapist is trained to gain difficult positions.

MONTHLY CONFERENCES

All therapists, teachers and medical social workers should meet regularly for discussion.

Holidays should be arranged if desired, to rest the parents, and to enlarge the child's experiences. Vocational assessment and training have to be considered. Parents should be put in touch with The Spastic Society (12 Park Crescent, London W.1).

THE SEVERELY DISABLED PATIENT

The home treatment as already described should be instituted with regular visits to the doctor and physiotherapist during the year. Improvement is usually slow and the treatment repetitive. Although the patient may develop only a few milestones, it is valuable to reduce spasticity so that he is more mobile. Thus, he is easier to look after, more comfortable, and safer in sitting as he will have some balance.

THE LIGHTLY HANDICAPPED CHILD

Spasticity and abnormal reflexes increase with effort; the effort of weight, speed or complexity. Abnormality must be elicited in these patients, in order to treat it. For instance, the hemiplegic arm and hand will become more spastic if the patient weight lifts with the good arm, or the patient may be able to dorsiflex his foot, but not if at the same time he flexes the hip and extends the knee as required in walking.

CONCLUSION

The spastic, athetoid patient with variable rigidity or ataxic patient all have abnormal reflex patterns of posture and movements. Therefore, all require basically reflex inhibiting postures. All are retarded in the development of their milestones, and, therefore, need training in postures, and in reflex and voluntary movements during inhibition.

In addition the spastic patient has hypertonus, which decreases in reflex inhibiting postures. The athetoid and variable rigidity patients have fluctuating muscle tone, and the ataxic patient low muscle tone: their movements are spoilt because of their defective postural background, and they require stabilising techniques.

If the physiotherapist fails to train the patient in normal patterns of posture and movement, the patient will not be able to do it for himself, because his efforts always pass down certain stereotyped nervous pathways, depending on the severity of his injury, and he can do nothing about it. In addition the treatment must be vigorous enough to be effective; thus the physiotherapist should work at a posture or movement not easily obtained, or should control a position in which the patient himself is able to achieve new activities. Every improvement in range, position, movement and power gained in a treatment will be more easily obtained the next time. The patient should feel neither pain nor discomfort.

Author's Note.

The Swedish splint is obtainable from Beckett and Bird, Ltd., 8 Bentinck St., London W.1.

For information about riding, application may be made to the Director, Riding Centre for the Disabled, Grange Farm, Chigwell, Essex.

CHAPTER 7

Virus Infections of the Nervous System

REVISED BY MARGARET POTTER, M.C.S.P.

ERTAIN VIRUSES HAVE A special affinity for the nervous system and are known as neurotropic viruses. These micro-organisms reach the brain and spinal cord by travelling along the axons of the cranial and spinal nerves; they invade the nerve cells, multiply within them and produce pathological changes.

Two main classes of lesion result; a non-suppurative inflammatory process, as in acute poliomyelitis, epidemic encephalitis and herpes zoster, and an encephalo-myelitis in which the primary lesion is a demyelination of nerve fibres.

ACUTE POLIOMYELITIS

This is an acute infectious disease which may be epidemic or sporadic. At one time known as infantile paralysis, it is not confined to children, although the one to five year age group is particularly vulnerable. Unlike many other diseases the healthy, active child or adult is most often affected.

The virus, of which several types have been isolated, is spread by patients or by carriers who do not necessarily develop clinically recognisable poliomyelitis. The virus has been isolated from the naso-pharynx and faeces, both in the pre- and post-paralytic stage. An attack by one type of virus does not immunise against the others—though the number of patients who have had poliomyelitis twice is very small.

Two vaccines are now available—'dead' by injection, and 'live' given orally. Since their use, the incidence of poliomyelitis has dropped dramatically.

PATHOLOGY

The virus enters the body through the naso-pharynx or the alimentary canal. It is thought to travel from the former to the brain stem via certain cranial nerves and from the latter via the intestines and sympathetic nerve fibres to the spinal cord.

The lesions produced by the virus have a definite distribution. In the spinal cord the lumbar enlargement is most often attacked and less commonly the cervical. The micro-organism has a special affinity for the anterior horn cells though posterior horn and posterior nerve root ganglion cells are also invaded. In the brain, the cells affected are usually those of the nuclei in mid-brain, pons and medulla. Occasionally the pyramidal cells of the motor area of the cortex are attacked and the meninges can also be affected.

Inflammatory, followed by degenerative, changes are produced. When these subside there is likely to be atrophy of the anterior horns in the affected area and secondary degeneration of the axons of the destroyed cells. In all but the abortive cases, in which necrosis of cells does not occur, muscular paralysis develops—the extent depending on the degree of cell damage.

CLINICAL COURSE

1. Pre-paralytic stage.
2. Acute paralytic stage.
3. Convalescent stage.
4. Residual stage.

These divisions are for simplification and it must be remembered that there is a certain amount of overlap. Treatment employed at each stage is discussed, but it must be emphasised that the clinical progress of the patient is the only guide to progression. The incubation period is variable, but is commonly seven to ten days. Infection lasts about six weeks.

PRE-PARALYTIC STAGE

This is the critical stage of the disease when the viruses are multiplying in the central nervous system. Muscle fatigue at this time invites a heavy attack on the anterior horn cells supplying these muscles. A typical case shows the features of a major illness with fever, headache, nausea and diarrhoea. Rigidity of the neck and spine is a characteristic feature, probably due to meningeal irritation. There is often pain in the back and legs accompanied by muscle tenderness. This could be due to involvement of the posterior roots and ganglia.

Treatment consists of bed rest and all precautions to prevent spread of infection.

ACUTE PARALYTIC STAGE

Development of the lower motor neurone paralysis is the hallmark of the disease. The muscles become flaccid and the deep reflexes are abolished. In most cases the paralysis is of rapid onset and asymmetrical.

The limbs continue tender to the touch and movement is painful and limited by the guarding spasm of muscles capable of contraction. It is thought that movement causes traction on sensitive nerves.

Respiratory complications are of major importance and the mortality rate is closely allied to the early recognition and treatment of the different types.

There are three main types of respiratory complication:

(1) *Bulbar* when the brain stem is attacked and the muscles of deglutition become paralysed leading to the pooling of saliva and inability to swallow. The secretions from mouth and nose may be inhaled.

The patient should be nursed prone with the head down and suction may be needed to remove salivary and bronchial secretions.

(2) *Spinal* with paralysis of the respiratory muscles and a resultant inability to maintain sufficient lung movement. Artificial aid may be necessary, given by cabinet respirator, cuirasse or rocking bed.

(3) *Bulbo-spinal* which is a combination of the above. Tracheotomy may be necessary, in which case an intermittent positive-pressure respirator is used.

Chest care: The patient's breathing can be helped by:

(a) Postural drainage.
(b) Gentle percussion and squeezing on expiration.
(c) Help with coughing.

It must be remembered that with respiratory poliomyelitis the most important aims are at variance. They are:

Rest to avoid further paralysis.
Positioning to avoid lung collapse.

The care of the chest, which is the life-saver, naturally has priority, but the patient must be handled gently and all unnecessary strain, mental as well as physical, avoided. Respiratory distress and paralysis are both terrifying symptoms and the staff dealing with these patients should be particularly kind, efficient and reassuring.

If the patient is in an iron lung little attention is necessary, though he should be turned from side to side as far as possible and the lung tilted.

After tracheotomy, when the patient is on an intermittent positive pressure respirator, there are nearly always secretions which can cause partial collapse of the lungs. By posturing all areas of the lung tissue are drained and this is helped by vibration, percussion and forced pushing on expiration in all positions. This routine is complicated by the fact that movement is frequently painful, pulls on the tracheotomy tube causing irritation and that until the inflatable tube in the trachea can be let down, the patient has no voice and is consequently difficult to understand. Frequent 'sucking-out' is necessary and this too can be painful and causes further irritation if done roughly. Co-operation between nursing and physiotherapy staff is essential.

For milder cases, being turned from side to side in the semi-prone position with the foot of the bed elevated about 10° is advocated for the majority of the time. There is a natural slope of 15° in the respiratory tract which must be remembered when doing postural drainage with the patient lying (25° tilt of the bed is needed to get 10° in the tract). With the patient in this position secretions can be eliminated either passively through the mouth or by coughing with or without aid from the physiotherapist.

General treatment

(1) Gentle passive movements carried just to the point of pain are started as soon as possible. Painful stretching is harmful as weakened or paralysed muscle can easily be torn and nerve roots damaged.

(2) Moist heat relieves pain and tenderness and hot packs can be given before movements.

(3) Contractures can develop through bad positioning in bed. All paralysed limbs should be comfortably supported to avoid stretching and prevent deformities. Change of position allows pressure points to be relieved as well as helping to prevent lung collapse, intestinal stasis, etc.

(4) Voluntary muscles should be charted, using the Medical Research Council 1-5 grading, when the patient has settled down. It may be done over a period of days to prevent overtiring.

Prognosis

This should be considered under recovery of muscle power and of muscle function.

(*a*) *Muscle Power.* Most muscles will, with treatment, recover approximately two grades on the correct charting at four to six weeks. The rate of recovery is most rapid the first six months, after which it progressively slows down. It is slower in adults than children. No increase in grade is expected after twenty-four months unless correction of a deformity allows a muscle to work at a better mechanical advantage. Ninety per cent of muscles that are completely paralysed at six months will remain so.

(*b*) *Muscle Function.* This will continue over a much longer period, in severe cases, independence may not be reached for several years, if ever, but co-ordination, confidence, endurance and skill will all be developed with help. Treatment should be continued as long as it helps to improve the locomotor or respiratory function, but not after it has ceased to do so.

CONVALESCENT STAGE

This period merges indefinitely with the preceding one and continues so long as there is functional recovery of the affected musculature. Modifications of rest and more active physiotherapy are allowed as the pain and tenderness, pyrexia and rigidity of neck and back disappear.

Some patients recover rapidly but, though allowed home, should be warned to take things very slowly and be given a progressive scheme of exercises to follow.

In respiratory and bulbar cases there is a limit to what can be done for the limbs—imposed partly by the need to deal with the chest and partly because the patients tire more easily.

Weaning from cabinet respirator

With the patient's co-operation, 'free breathing' is started as soon as possible. The tank is opened and the physiotherapist compresses the patient's chest encouraging him to take over alone. It is essential:

(1) to return the patient to aid *before* he gets tired, or
(2) immediately he indicates the need.

Refusing aid at this time will only cause fear and loss of confidence. It is better to increase these periods without the use of alternate aid if possible. When the patient can breathe freely for about half an hour, he can be lifted on to a comfortable bed. The first few times the patient feels happier if someone is around to put him back when he feels the need. The final stage of weaning is learning to sleep without help. The patient must be assured that he will not stop breathing if he sleeps and that though he will only sleep lightly and not for long at first, this will not hurt him. It is usual to try one night out and then two or three nights in the tank. The day's programme before his night out should be cut to avoid fatigue, or he will not sleep so well. Where the need for aid is likely to be prolonged, help from a cuirasse, rocking bed or positive pressure belt may be given.

Weaning from intermittent positive-pressure respirator

'Free breathing' is encouraged as before, the cuff deflated for longer periods and eventually, if recovery is good, the point reached where a small uncuffed tube can be inserted and the respirator not used. With a more severely affected patient, alternative aid would be given instead of the intermittent positive-pressure respirator. There are a very few patients whose chests are so productive that it is not advisable to close the stoma.

Where closure is going ahead, it is advisable to accustom the patient to another form of artificial respirator which can be used to help him over the week or so while the stoma is closing. The tube is removed and strapping applied. Plastic surgery is recommended later for cosmesis. Throughout this period, chest physiotherapy is given as indicated. It should be preventative as well as aimed at clearing the chest, so postural drainage becomes a routine. The patient and physiotherapist learn the 'feel' of the chest very quickly and can usually judge fairly accurately the whereabouts of secretions. Unnecessary 'pushing' and 'sucking-out' can cause irritation and produce secretions so treatment must be a balance between too little and too much.

RE-EDUCATION

It cannot be stressed too much in the treatment of poliomyelitis that ingenuity and the adaptation of accepted techniques are the real skill and the personality of the physiotherapist plays as great a part as the apparatus she uses.

(1) *Movements in bed*

(a) Passive: active assisted: free: resisted.

(b) Proprioceptive facilitation techniques.

(c) Use of slings and springs in which to suspend arms to obtain greater function.

(2) *Pool therapy*

The design of pools varies. Ideally there should be facility for patients to do exercises in lying and in sitting and reasonable lengths at variable depths, with handrails, in which they can learn to walk. The water should be heated to between 90–98° F. (32–37° C.) according to the amount of activity possible. The buoyancy makes possible active exercises which could not be performed on dry land. All ranges of movement of affected joints are encouraged—a head sling and rubber rings, or the like, to support the moving limbs being the only essential apparatus. Trick movements should not be encouraged until there is no hope of further recovery. This necessitates careful fixation of other joints by the physiotherapist. By changing the position of the patient in the water most muscle groups can be worked through three progressions. That is using the water:

(a) to assist movement.

(b) only as a support (neutral).

(c) to resist movement.

Patients progress from lying to sitting, balancing, standing, walking and going up steps according to their rate of recovery and their ability to master the various stages.

(3) *Slings, pulleys and springs*

Suspension exercises again are aimed at increasing mobility and strengthening muscle power by using Guthrie-Smith frames or home-made versions.

(4) *Mat exercises*

Much work can be done on mats placed ideally on a raised platform beside which the physiotherapist can stand. In addition to general exercises, proprioceptive facilitation techniques, etc., the patient can be taught to roll over, press up on his arms, balance in sitting (with a mirror in front) and even to kneel and crawl.

(5) *Ambulation*

From walking in the pool the patient progresses to walking between parallel bars in the gymnasium and eventually, when possible, to crutches, sticks or walking aids. Calipers may be used if one or both legs are rail, but the weight of the apparatus can defeat its purpose. A supporting belt may be necessary if there is trunk involvement.

Balancing is the first stage, then weight transference and finally a step is taken.

RESIDUAL STAGE

This stage is reached when no new muscle recovery is seen. Treatment is now aimed at improving the functioning muscles to enable them to do their work better and, where possible, take over from paralysed ones.

Surgery may be contemplated and, though not usually performed until later, the surgeon may order certain muscles to be treated prior to transplant.

If walking proves impracticable, life must be tackled in a chair and the patient taught to use one to the best advantage.

Slow progress usually continues over a matter of years, the patient learning the knack of doing more and more for himself. It is sometimes difficult to persuade a patient that treatment has served its purpose and that his energies must be used to develop his own way of doing things at home or at work, but this is often an essential part of 'treatment'. Home visits to advise on modifications in the house should be made by the physiotherapist as well as the occupational therapist and medical social worker where disablement is severe. Long periods of out-patient treatment should be discouraged.

Children should be checked at an orthopaedic clinic routinely every few months so that developing deformities can be stopped if possible, or at least measures taken to control them.

HERPES ZOSTER

Herpes zoster gives an acute vesicular eruption in the cutaneous distribution of any sensory nerve root.

The condition is an acute infection of the posterior nerve root ganglion of the spinal cord, the trigeminal or the geniculate ganglia.

The changes are those of acute inflammation in the affected ganglion, with hyperaemia, swelling and tiny haemorrhages.

The condition usually commences with a brief febrile illness lasting a few days. During this period fairly severe pain is experienced in the area in which the cutaneous eruption will appear. A few days later erythema occurs in this area, followed by the formation of vesicles. The vesicles are filled with clear fluid and the skin around is erythematous and swollen. About the fifth or sixth day from the time of eruption the vesicles dry up and scabs are formed, these tend to fall off leaving tiny scars or pigmented areas. Very occasionally the infection appears to spread across the cord and involve the motor cells and fibres. In this case a paralysis of muscles supplied by this segment of the cord will occur, with loss of tone, diminished or lost deep reflexes and disturbances in circulation.

There is an interesting connection between herpes zoster and chickenpox, and it is not unusual to find that an attack of the former condition in one person may be followed by chickenpox in another person in contact with the first.

OUTLINE OF TREATMENT BY PHYSIOTHERAPY

It is not very often that the physiotherapist is called in to help in the treatment of these cases. It may be to deal with the muscular paralysis should this occur. If this is so then physiotherapy will be given on the lines indicated for a case of acute poliomyelitis. On the other hand, ultraviolet light may be ordered for its counter-irritant effect in the case of a post-herpetic neuralgia, when a second degree erythema should be obtained in the area of eruption. Ultra-violet light sometimes proves very effective in preventing or eliminating neuralgia but in other cases it may have no effect at all.

ENCEPHALITIS LETHARGICA

This is an inflammatory condition of the brain thought to be caused by a virus which produces degeneration of nerve cells particularly in the basal ganglion and brain stem. The residual symptoms closely resemble those of Parkinson's disease and should be treated similarly.

POST-INFECTIVE ENCEPHALITIS

An acute widely disseminated encephalo-myelitis occasionally develops as a sequel to one of the infectious diseases of virus origin, particularly measles. Few cases reach the physiotherapy department as spontaneous recovery is usual. If Parkinsonism, hemiplegia, etc., do develop they should be treated as such.

CHAPTER 8

Muscular Atrophies

REVISED BY ROSEMARY SMITH, M.C.S.P.

THE PRESENCE OF MUSCULAR ATROPHY is a familiar feature to most physiotherapists. If atrophy due to disuse is omitted, the many other varieties may be classified into five main groups readily recognisable, if such factors as age and method of onset, distribution and type of atrophy are considered.

These groups are:

Motor Neurone Disease.
Peroneal Muscular Atrophy.
Arthritic Atrophy.
Muscular Dystrophy.

In addition, syringomyelia leads to muscular atrophy, though sensory and trophic symptoms are also present.

MOTOR NEURONE DISEASE

The pathological process in all types of motor neurone disease is a primary degeneration of the lower or upper motor neurones or both. The cause of this degeneration is unknown, the origin is not inflammatory nor is there an accompanying inflammatory reaction. It first appears about middle life. All types are characterised by progressive wasting and therefore weakness, by fasciculation, by the bilateral nature of the condition and by the fact that electrical reactions are usually at first normal but gradually the response weakens as atrophy progresses. In the later stages the reaction of degeneration will be present.

There are three main areas of the central nervous system which appear to be affected by the progressive degenerative pathological process, and for this reason they used to be described as three different diseases, viz:

(i) Progressive muscular atrophy when lower motor neurone lesions predominate.

(ii) Progressive bulbar palsy when muscles innervated from the medulla are first involved.

(iii) Amyotrophic lateral sclerosis when pyramidal lesions are combined with lower motor neurone lesions.

Clinically all the cases show progressive muscle wasting and fasciculation usually beginning in the small muscles of the hand, or in the tongue and lips whose muscles are innervated from the medulla. Symptoms of a pyramidal lesion causing muscular spasticity may also occur.

The more widespread the fasciculation the more serious is the outlook.

OUTLINE OF PHYSIOTHERAPY

No form of treatment as yet known arrests the progress of motor neurone disease, therefore physical measures cannot hope to do a great deal for the patient, yet cases of amyotrophic lateral sclerosis do reach the department of physical medicine. A certain amount of improvement may temporarily occur because it is possible that hypertrophy of unaffected motor units may take place, giving greater strength to the affected muscles. The development of deformities may be prevented and the circulation and nutrition of the muscles and limb as a whole improved. In this condition, unlike poliomyelitis, gross circulatory changes do not occur but in advanced cases the limb is likely to be cold and stiff due to lack of use. Above all, physiotherapy has a definite psychological value. As long as the patient is receiving treatment he does not feel that he is a hopeless case; thus he remains cheerful and co-operative. The physical measures chosen to aid these patients must be carefully selected. They do not follow the lines set out in Chapter 3 p. 151 because the disease is progressive and fatigue might hasten the degenerative processes in the spinal cord. Therefore two points must be considered: firstly, physical measures must not tire the patient and, secondly, they must not be unduly stimulating. For this reason electrical stimulation and difficult exercises are to be avoided. Careful active exercise may be employed to retain present strength or even slightly to improve it, but it must be well within the patient's capabilities and below the point of fatigue.

It may be noticed that, throughout, work for all four limbs is advocated. This is because the condition will progress in spite of treatment but it is just possible that progress might be delayed by maintaining the condition of the muscles.

PERONEAL MUSCULAR ATROPHY
(Charcot-Marie-Tooth type)

This type of muscular atrophy resembles motor neurone disease in that it is due to degeneration of nerve cells.

The cause of the condition is unknown but it appears to be transmitted directly from one of the parents and its onset occurs in the young adult.

The changes are those of degeneration in the anterior horn of the lumbar enlargement and in the anterior nerve roots. In addition, unlike the other types, the posterior columns may show degenerative changes. Wasting and weakness begin in the plantar muscles of the feet, spread to the peronei and to extensors longus digitorum and hallucis, later affecting the calf muscles and the lower third of the quadriceps group. This peculiar distribution leads to the development of deformities, particularly to a severe pes cavus and foot drop. The wasting of the lower third of the quadriceps gives a peculiar appearance to the thigh resembling that of a bottle.

The ankle jerk will be diminished and gradually lost as wasting of the calf muscles progresses. Fasciculation is often seen in the wasting muscles but it is not a constant feature. Electrical reactions remain normal but are weaker than usual.

Considerable impairment of all forms of sensation in the affected area may be present and diminished position sense may give rise to ataxia.

Occasionally a similar condition may occur in the hands and distal one-third of the forearms. In few cases does the lesion progress beyond the lower third of thigh and forearm; it usually arrests spontaneously at this level. Since progress does not occur beyond this point the disease is not fatal. It leaves the patient with a certain amount of disability, but it is surprising how slight this disability actually is. There will be a foot drop but this can be adequately dealt with.

Since the condition will cease to progress, the essential feature is to try to prevent the development of permanent deformities and to maintain as much muscle power as possible. The prevention of trophic disturbances and skin lesions is also an important point. Physiotherapy will therefore prove beneficial. Any form of heat should be carefully applied owing to the defective sensibility. Passive movements are particularly important to prevent contracture of plantar fascia, plantar muscles and tendo achillis and to retain mobility in the toes and foot. Careful active work to maintain reasonable strength in all affected muscles may be given.

ARTHRITIC ATROPHY

This type of atrophy is not directly due to lesions of the nervous system, but probably only to disuse.

Atrophy of muscle is usually obvious in all types of arthritic conditions. It differs from other types of atrophy in its distribution since it occurs only in those muscles which are acting on the affected joints.

P

Not only does it occur in these groups but it is also most marked in the extensor muscles proximal to the joint; thus, for example, in arthritis of the knee joint the quadriceps group is more severely atrophied than the hamstring muscles, while in a lesion of the wrist joint the dorsiflexors of the wrist are more affected than the flexors. Wasting of the muscle fibres reduces their power with the result that it may be impossible to obtain a full range of extension in the joint, and flexion deformities may develop. A true fasciculation is not associated with this type of atrophy but muscles may be tender on pressure. Electrical reaction will remain qualitatively unchanged but responses will be weaker. Deep reflexes will be present but diminished in strength.

Prevention may be difficult. Static exercises give the best chance of success when the arthritis is active and the joints therefore need rest. Treatment can only be successful if active work is given for the muscles, but it must be carefully graded.

MUSCULAR DYSTROPHY

In cases of primary muscular disease, no demonstrable change in the nervous system is present. The disease is one in which some congenital defect in the muscle is probably present and pathological changes take place without known cause. Different types of muscular dystrophy occur but certain features are characteristic of all cases.

There is a strong heredo-familial incidence, the disease being most often transmitted to the males of the family through unaffected females. The age at which symptoms first appear is earlier than in other muscular atrophies, being either in infancy, childhood or adolescence. Unlike other muscular atrophies, muscles are often enlarged because increase in the connective tissue of the muscles occurs at the same time as atrophy of the muscle fibres. Fasciculation is never seen, neither are the muscles tender on pressure. The electrical reactions remain qualitatively normal though their strength diminishes as power wanes. Tendon reflexes, which at first are normal, gradually diminish and are eventually lost. The distribution of atrophy also differs; instead of affecting the distal segments of the limbs or the muscles of speech, deglutition and respiration, this lesion attacks the limb girdles and the muscles of expression.

The pathological changes occur in the muscle fibres and in the connective tissue of the muscles. In the early stages the fibres are swollen and the nuclei increase in numbers, later the fibres undergo atrophy. Meanwhile the interstitial tissue increases in quantity and fat is deposited within it. According as to which process is most advanced, so the actual muscle increases or decreases in size. Whether atrophy or hypertrophy predomin-ate, loss of power invariably occurs and hypertrophy is thus a pseudo-, not a true, hypertrophy.

Muscular dystrophies are classed into three varieties, according to the muscles affected and the age of onset: pseudo-hypertrophic type, Erb's juvenile type and the facio-scapulo-humeral type.

Pseudo-hypertrophic muscular dystrophy. This is the most common variety. It attacks young boys and makes its first appearance in infancy. Certain muscles show hypertrophy while others are atrophied. Pseudo-hypertrophy occurs in the calf muscles, quadriceps and glutei, in the lower part of sacro-spinalis and in the deltoids and spinati. Atrophy is seen in the flexors and adductors of the hips and the hamstring muscles, while in the upper extremities the biceps and triceps are sometimes affected; the lower part of trapezius, pectoralis major and serratus anterior are also involved. The result of these changes is a weakness of some movements and the development of deformities. An increasing disability in stance and gait gradually manifests itself. The child whose extensors are weakened and flexors shortened will have a marked lordosis in standing since the pelvic tilt will be increased and the trunk will be thrown back to compensate. Weakness of abductors will cause a waddling gait. A tendency to clumsy walking and liability to fall easily, with difficulty in negotiating stairs, will be early symptoms. As the condition progresses, a characteristic rise from the supine position is noticeable and even diagnostic. If the child is placed on his back and then asked to get up, he first rolls over onto his face then gets onto his hands and knees, the hands are then placed on the thighs and he works his way up, by pushing against the thighs, to erect position, finally achieving it by jerking the trunk backwards. The atrophy of the shoulder girdle muscles results in inability to depress the arms against resistance so that if the child is picked up he slides through the physio-therapist's hands. Elevation of the arms is reduced, there is absence of the anterior axillary folds, the scapulae are winged and rotate so that the glenoid cavities tend to face downwards. The shoulders fall forward.

The mother's attention is often drawn to the child's condition by the enlargement of the calves and the late attempt to walk or the clumsy gait. In time the connective tissue tends to shorten and, as the calf muscles contract, the child will stand and walk on the toes.

The condition progresses until the child is unable to get about at all; usually he does not attain adult life, as lack of activity and atrophy of pectoral muscles predisposes towards respiratory affections.

Erb's juvenile type. This type appears rather later, usually in adolescence or in early adult life. There is much less often hypertrophy, atrophy being the outstanding feature. The shoulder girdle is affected first and most severely though the pelvic girdle is affected later. Particularly noticeable is the atrophy of trapezius, pectoralis major and serratus anterior, giving rise to the deformity of winging of the scapulae, and resulting in great difficulty in elevating the arms, through abduction or flexion, above shoulder level.

This condition progresses very much more slowly than the previous type and the prognosis is therefore more favourable.

Facio-scapulo-humeral variety. This appears rather earlier than Erb's type but later than the pseudo-hypertrophic variety. Both boys and girls are affected, and the progress is more rapid. There is a similar condition of the shoulder girdle but, as the name implies, the facial muscles are also involved. The orbicularis oris muscle is usually hypertrophied, so that the lips are thick and everted and the child is unable to close them properly. Drinking and whistling are difficult and speech is not clear. Atrophy of the other facial muscles gives a peculiar mournful expression to the face and closure of the eyelids becomes defective.

Eventually the muscles of the pelvic girdle may also be attacked and posture and gait resemble that of the first variety.

OUTLINE OF TREATMENT BY PHYSICAL MEASURES

Since all these conditions are progressive and for none is there a cure, physical measures are relatively ineffective. The main purpose is to keep the child up and about a little longer than might otherwise be possible. This may be done by preventing the development of permanent deformities such as flexion contracture of the hip joints, shortening of the calf muscles, and pes cavus, and by maintaining the nutrition of the affected muscle groups. The development of respiratory diseases may also be delayed by the use of physical measures. Breathing exercises and a light general scheme of exercises may be given to aid circulation and maintain freedom of joints of the limbs and trunk.

An attempt should be made to delay lateral curvature of the spine and its consequent sequelae by wearing light but rigid spinal support.

As in motor neurone disease, care must be taken not to fatigue muscles as this may accelerate the process.

AMYOTONIA CONGENITA

This should not be discussed under the heading of muscular atrophies, since atrophy is not a characteristic feature, but since it is a primary muscular disease it bears a close relationship to the preceding conditions and will therefore be described at this point. It is a condition of lack of tone in the voluntary muscles noticed soon after birth or in early infancy following some illness. The muscles are small and soft though not atrophied. They fail to harden in contraction and their power is so slight that the child may be unable to hold up its head, sit up or walk. Reflexes are diminished and the electrical reactions show a weak normal response.

Unlike the other disorders no progression occurs; in fact, over a long period some slight improvement takes place and in time the child may learn to sit up, though without apparatus he may never attain sufficient strength to stand or walk. One danger is that of damage to joints since muscular atonia will allow them to be carried far beyond their normal range, hence grotesque postures can easily be taken up. A second complication is that of contracture. If the infant is unable to stand, he may be propped up in the sitting position and adaptive shortening of the flexors of the hips and knees may occur.

Because of the possibility of improvement, physical treatment is definitely of value. By careful passive movements contractures should be prevented or tissues may be gently stretched if these have already occurred. The nutrition of the muscles may be increased by a light general massage and active exercises may help to speed up the natural improvement of muscle tone and strength. The child can be taught by gradual stages to hold up its head and to sit up unsupported. If this stage is satisfactorily reached, the next step is to gain the standing position and independent walking. For this the use of weight-bearing calipers attached to a light trunk support may be found possible. It is part of the physiotherapist's work to train the child to stand and walk in the apparatus and to teach the mother how to apply it and keep it in good condition. A reasonably good result is likely to be obtained if the child does not succumb to some intercurrent infection.

MYASTHENIA GRAVIS

This also is not a condition of muscular atrophy but it is a condition in which muscular power is weakened without apparent change in the nervous system and for this reason it is described with other primary muscular disorders.

The condition affects women more often than men and the first symptoms are usually seen in early adult life, though it does occasionally appear in the middle-aged. It is characterised by absence of muscular atrophy while at the same time there is rapid fatigue, and inability to contract voluntary muscles.

The cause is unknown but it is thought that acetyl-choline, normally liberated at the motor-end plate, transmitting the nerve impulse to the muscle fibre, is either not liberated or is destroyed too rapidly. The result of this is a weakened muscular contraction. It is quite often found in these patients that a large thymus gland is still present; in fact removal of this gland has been found to have a beneficial effect upon the condition, in some patients.

There is considerable variability in the onset of the symptoms in myasthenia gravis. In some cases, only the muscles innervated by the brain stem are affected, in others limb and trunk musculature is also involved. In the first case the patient finds that as the day goes on she has difficulty in keeping the eyes open and she has to tilt the head back to compensate for the ptosis. Mastication may become increasingly difficult throughout the day; the head may tend to fall forward and the patient may be seen in a characteristic posture, sitting with the chin supported in the hands and the eyes propped open by the fingers. Squint, diplopia, difficulty in speech and deglutition may all be present from time to time.

When the limbs are affected the patient may find increasing difficulty in lifting the arms, in walking or remaining erect at all.

It is difficult to give any prognosis since so much variation occurs. Some cases progress rapidly until they are unable to perform any voluntary action and they may die from failure of the respiratory muscles or disturbance of deglutition. Others may undergo complete arrest while yet others follow a slow chronic course. Temporary improvement for a few hours is obtained by the use of prostigmine but this does not provide a permanent cure. As has already been pointed out improvement is gained in some cases by thymectomy.

As the disease is characterised by relapses and remissions, during the myasthenic crises complete bed rest is essential in the hope of remission occurring. Physiotherapy may be called for to carry out routine chest care and the patient may have to undergo tracheotomy and artificial respiration. These crises can occasionally be precipitated by neostigmine poisoning.

SYRINGOMYELIA

Though many other symptoms occur in this chronic disease of the spinal cord, muscular atrophy is a constant and outstanding sign and for this reason the condition is dealt with in this chapter. The disease attacks both men and women equally, in adolescence or early adult life, and its cause is unknown.

The essential feature is a proliferation of the neuroglial tissue in the grey commissure and base of the posterior horn of the spinal cord in the dorsal and lower cervical segments. The newly formed glial tissue gradually softens and liquefies and, as it is removed by phagocytosis, long cavities remain. Sometimes the lesion remains confined to the upper dorsal region, in other cases it appears to spread along the whole length of the cord.

The symptoms of the lesion are the result of pressure and destruction and depend on the extent of the lesion. The first symptoms are usually sensory due to pressure on, or destruction of, the sensory fibres conveying painful and thermal stimuli as they cross in the grey commissure to reach the opposite side of the cord. A dissociated anaesthesia arises since light touch, postural and vibration senses are unimpaired. The patient suffers from diminished or lost ability to appreciate thermal or painful stimuli. Consequently scars and ulcers are likely to be seen on the fingers and Charcot's joints may develop. The shoulder joint is most often attacked and is liable to be completely disorganised, since lost pain sensation will allow severe trauma without awareness of damage. As the condition progresses the anterior horn becomes involved and damage to the motor cells will result in a progressive weakness and wasting commencing in the small muscles of one or both hands and spreading in a similar manner to the progress of a progressive muscular atrophy. Very rarely does complete paralysis occur and the patient often retains a surprising amount of use in the hands. Deformities, particularly claw hand, are likely to develop. If the lesion spreads laterally the lateral horn will be involved in the process with involvement of the pre-ganglionic sympathetic fibres. Circulatory disturbances will then arise, the hands become cyanosed and puffy, the skin thin and shiny, the subcutaneous tissues are thickened so that the hand feels soft and boneless to the touch.

A further lateral spread may cause pressure on the lateral columns and spasticity of the legs will then occur.

Physiotherapy is nearly always ordered, its object being to prevent deformities, improve the circulation and to bring about hypertrophy of unaffected fibres of the wasted muscles. The treatment therefore resembles that of progressive muscular atrophy but since progress is slower there is not quite the same danger of fatigue and the treatment may often be slightly progressed instead of regressed as in the former case.

CHAPTER 9

Traumatic Lesions of the Spinal Cord

REVISED BY F. McILWRAITH, M.C.S.P.

THE TREATMENT OF traumatic lesions of the spinal cord causing paraplegia or tetraplegia is essentially a matter of very close teamwork between the doctor, nursing staff, physiotherapist, occupational therapist, social worker, the patient and the patient's relatives.

Causes. Dislocation of one or more vertebrae, with or without fracture of the vertebral body, resulting in either complete trans-section of the spinal cord, or crushing of the spinal cord with paralysis of the body below that level.

Aims of treatment. Adaptation to life in a wheelchair and return to a normal and useful life as soon as possible. This is achieved by readjustment of the neuro-muscular system, re-education of bladder and bowels and psychological rehabilitation.

Assessment. The physiotherapist should be present at the doctor's examination of the patient to be acquainted with the type of fracture and/or dislocation and the level and degree of the neurological lesion. The physiotherapist must also know whether the spinal cord injury is associated with other injuries such as fractured ribs, skull, etc. Furthermore, the previous medical history should be taken into consideration, especially whether there is or has been any chronic chest condition or any other internal illness.

Level of Lesion. The amount of damage done is governed by the part of the spinal cord which has been severed or crushed, i.e. cervical, thoracic or lumbar portions, and in cauda equina lesions whether anterior and posterior roots are involved.

Recording. A careful record is made of all paralysed or impaired muscles, the assessment being in the form of the Medical Research Council's 0 to 5 grading. It is important that this record be kept up during the patient's stay in hospital so that any change may be noticed and the information available when necessary.

Stage I—in bed

The vital factor in this stage is position. The patient is nursed with the spine in hyperextension; a patient with dislocation of a cervical spine may have skeletal traction to reduce the dislocation, and a patient with lumbar dislocation may have a firm pillow or roll at the site of the dislocation, when lying supine, to reduce the dislocation.

To avoid pressure sores, the recently injured patient is nursed on the Egerton turning bed, his position being changed every two hours from supine to side-lying and then returned to supine. In each position he has at least two pillows between his legs to maintain abduction of the hips and prevent pressure on the medial surface of the knees and ankles. A tetraplegic patient will have a sponge or foam rubber pad strapped to each hand to maintain the functional position of the hand, with abduction of the thumb and semi-flexion of the fingers. Once a day the patient is lifted completely from the bed by a trained nurse. The extended position of the spine is maintained throughout and traction of the neck is maintained where necessary. No flexion or rotation of the spine is allowed at any level.

More chronic lesions may be nursed on pack beds and turned less frequently, but constant attention is still given to pressure areas, the onus of skin care gradually being transferred to the patient.

Breathing exercises

The patient initially will be suffering from shock, with consequent shallow respiration, and any lesion above Thoracic 5 will have impaired respiration due to paralysis of the abdominal muscles and intercostal muscles. Those with cervical lesions at and above Cervical 5 will have great difficulty in breathing, due to paralysis or paresis of the diaphragm and these patients will often need a tracheostomy. All patients should be given breathing exercises as soon as possible, with special care of those with fractured ribs. Assistance may be given to tetraplegics by firm pressure on the lateral aspects of the thorax and upward pressure on the abdominal wall to press the abdominal contents against the diaphragm, timed carefully with the patient's natural expiration. These should be given several times a day and if necessary during the night. If any infection is suspected, the patient should be treated after every turn, with vibrations and assistance with coughing. Pressure on the abdominal wall may be used to assist a quadriplegic to cough, again timed with the patient's attempt to cough. This is also very helpful in assisting a tetraplegic to blow his nose, and often a chest infection can be avoided by keeping the nasal passages clear. If a chest infection does develop and the above treatment is insufficient, postural drainage and percussion may be given at the discretion of the doctor, especial care being taken in the case of a cervical lesion on traction, support being given to his shoulders and neck while the physiotherapist is percussing, to prevent any slipping down the bed due to the bed being raised.

With early prophylactic treatment, tracheostomy is rarely needed but if performed, the patient is treated in a similar way with assisted breathing exercises and coughing, and the sputum is then sucked out.

Passive movements

Treatment is begun immediately, to prevent contractures, promote circulation and prevent loss of elasticity in muscles. Every joint in the paralysed limbs is put through full range of movement at least once or twice every day. Overstretching of the muscles and joints must be avoided. An important point to remember is that many muscles pass over more than one joint and it is insufficient to stretch a muscle or muscle group by moving only one of these joints, e.g. in exercising the finger flexors, the wrist and elbow must be extended, as well as the interphalangeal joints. The patient should be treated while lying on his side, as well as while supine, to obtain the necessary extension of the hip joint and flexion of the knee, also to put the quadriceps muscle through full range of movement.

In addition, each joint must be moved carefully and rhythmically not less than twenty times in each direction of which the joint is capable, to promote circulation by the alternate stretching and relaxing of the walls of the vessels passing over the joints. This should be done twice a day.

Contra-indications. In lumbar and low thoracic lesions, the amount of hip flexion allowed is at the discretion of the doctor, as no flexion must occur at the affected intervertebral joints; however, hip flexion should be increased later, at the advice of the doctor, so that 90° is obtained by the time the patient is ready to start sitting up. In tetraplegias, elevation of the shoulder must be specially carefully performed, with the physiotherapist supporting above the shoulder to ensure that gleno-humeral movement only occurs and no movement in the neck.

All passive movements should be performed with great care, smoothly and without forcing or giving traction. The patient should be aware of the movement and watch, where possible, and should be instructed to try to join in actively, to retain the pattern of movement and knowledge of how to perform it.

Precautions. If a patient has not stood for some time he may have some osteoporosis and extra care must be taken to avoid any possibility of a fracture occurring.

Active Movements

The patient is encouraged to use his unaffected limbs as soon as possible, always avoiding rotation and flexion of the spine. A patient with a thoracic or lower lesion is given a chest expander as soon as allowed by the doctor, and instructed to use this ten to fifteen times every half hour. This must be carefully taught, to avoid rotation of the spine, and the optimum spring strength discovered. This exercise promotes circulation and strengthens transverse back, shoulder girdle, elbow and wrist extensor and hand muscles.

All impaired muscles and those showing signs of returning power are watched carefully and a record kept of any change. The patient is encouraged to exercise these himself during the day, as well as during his daily treatment. Resisted exercises may be given at the discretion of the doctor, as the muscles progress. Proprioceptive neuromuscular facilitation techniques are used extensively in cervical and incomplete lesions.

Electrical treatment

Faradic or galvanic stimulation may be given to impaired muscle groups and those innervated at the level of the lesion and expected to return. Especial care must be taken because of the impairment of sensation, and the method used is 'stroking' of the whole of the skin covering the muscle group, from one insertion to the other, so that neither electrode remains still for more than a few seconds, and the whole bulk of the muscle is included in the treatment. Not less than 600 stimulations must be given at each treatment.

Stage II—sitting up

When the fracture and/or dislocation is stable and the doctor gives permission for the patient to sit up, he is carefully raised to a sitting position. A tetraplegic will only be raised a few degrees for a few moments, because of the impairment in the sympathetic control and respiration. An abdominal support may be given to counteract the effects of the change of position causing hypotension, and it is important that the physiotherapist be present at this time to give assistance with breathing. A collar will be fitted before the patient is raised to prevent any flexion or rotation in the cervical spine and to support the head.

A paraplegic will be fitted with a spinal supporting corset for some time to avoid any possibility of re-dislocation and, according to the level of his lesion, will be able to maintain the upright position for fifteen minutes to half an hour.

The time is gradually increased each day and when the patient can sit upright comfortably for two hours, he is raised twice a day.

No passive movements may be given while the patient is sitting but active movements are encouraged, to assist circulation and begin retraining balance.

Stage III—in chair

When permitted by the doctor, the patient is lifted into a wheelchair which is provided with a four-inch foam rubber cushion. A tetraplegic patient will maintain this position for a few minutes—if necessary with his feet raised, and a patient with a lower lesion for about half an hour. He is taught to lift himself, to relieve pressure, for two minutes each ten minutes or quarter hour; a paraplegic should lift until his arms are fully extended with his hands on the arms of his chair, and a tetraplegic will learn to lean to one side and then the other and forward, but until he can do this, he must be lifted by one of the staff.

Balance exercises. As soon as the patient can sit in the chair for two hours and when the doctor gives permission, he is taken to a mirror of suitable height and taught to maintain an upright position. A tetraplegic is taught to use the weight of his arms to change his position, and a lower lesion is taught to sit straight unsupported while moving his arms forward, sideways and overhead. The mirror is used at first, so that he can use his sight to compensate for loss of sensation; then he is taught to balance without the mirror.

When his balance is good, the patient is taught to wheel the chair and to control it. A tetraplegic will need leather guards for the palms of his hands to protect the skin where there is loss of sensation and to provide greater friction against the tyres.

Stage IV—in the Department

When permission is granted, the patient is taken to the department. Latissimus dorsi exercises are given by pulling weights attached to ropes passing over ceiling pulleys, by means of handles attached to the other ends of the ropes, the weights being adjusted to the patient's ability. This is an important exercise, for the latissimus dorsi is innervated at C. 6, 7, 8 and is attached to the shoulder girdle and the pelvis, so that with the shoulder fixed it can raise the pelvis on that side and lift the leg off the floor, or with both sides working, both feet may be lifted.

Balance is taught with the patient sitting on a plinth, on a pillow, with his feet supported so that knees and hips are at right angles and thighs fully supported, and a mirror in front of him. The physiotherapist stands behind him ready to prevent him falling and instructs him in maintaining a good posture first with one arm lifted, then with two, then with his arms stretched forwards, sideways and upwards. When this is perfect, he goes through the same routine with his eyes closed.

Standing. When his sitting balance is perfect and the doctor's permission obtained, plaster of Paris back slabs are made, to maintain the patient's knees in extension, especial care being taken to avoid any ridges or sharp edges which might cause pressure, and the patient then stands between parallel bars with the plasters bandaged on firmly, and toe-springs fixed from below the knees to his shoes. A mirror is placed at the other end of the bars and balance exercises are given, teaching the patient to maintain a good posture while holding first with two hands, then with one. Then a step is attempted, using the latissimus dorsi if the side, hip and trunk flexors are paralysed, lifting both feet off the floor by pressing down on the bars and lifting the pelvis, extending his hips immediately his feet land on the floor. Swing-to gait is taught first, then four-point and finally swing-through for the lower lesions. He practises turning, sideways travelling and walking backwards and getting out of and into the chair.

A tetraplegic will only be able to stand for a minute or two at first, until the circulation has compensated for the impairment in control. To stand a tetraplegic, the physiotherapist brings him to the front of the chair, raises his hips up and forwards, keeping his shoulder back, making sure his feet do not slide forwards. She then moves behind him, holding him in the erect position while she does so. With one of her feet between his, she can then control any side flexion; with her arms under his shoulders and her hands in front of his shoulders, she can prevent flexion of spine and hips. The patient's hands are placed on the bars with the elbows fully extended, and he gradually learns to take his weight through his arms and maintain his balance and posture. When this has been achieved, he attempts movement by hitching his pelvis with the latissimus dorsi.

Functional Activities

A tetraplegic is given any gadgets necessary to permit him to feed himself while he is in bed, such as a fork with a large handle and a strap over his hand, a mug with a large handle into which he can hook his thumb, and so on.

As soon as the injured joint is stable and flexion is permitted, the patient starts learning to dress, wash, turn in bed, get from wheelchair to plinth and back and onto and off the bed and from chair to toilet and back, using an overhead pulley if necessary. A tetraplegic may need such gadgets as loops on socks or stockings and zips, elastic laces in shoes, a buttonhook, etc.

Care of skin.

Great stress is laid at all times on the need for great care in the prevention of sores due to the impairment of sensation; the patient is taught never to rest any denervated part on a hard surface, to watch for hot or sharp objects with which he might come in contact, never to try hot water with innervated skin, never to use hot-water bottles, to avoid having wrinkles in clothes, especially socks and pants and so on.

Stage V—out and about

When the patient is proficient in standing and walking unaided in the bars, the doctor may order calipers to be made for him. These are non-weight-bearing, with a hinge at the knee joint to allow him to sit in the chair, and must fit well, with no pressure anywhere, and with as few fastenings as possible, so that he can put them on for himself.

He learns to walk with elbow crutches, first with one crutch and one bar, inside the parallel bars, then with two crutches, starting from the beginning again with standing balance, lifting first one then the other crutch while maintaining his balance, with the physiotherapist standing behind him, ready to catch him if necessary. He then practises swing-to gait with two crutches, learning to lift his feet off the ground and place them down accurately, and then progresses to four-point gait and, for lower lesions, swing-through, when it is especially important for him to maintain hip extension while bringing his crutches forward, as flexion will cause him to 'jack-knife', owing to lack of control of hip extensors, and he will fall. He then practises walking on slopes and over uneven ground.

Standing from the wheelchair with two crutches may be achieved in two ways:

1. Patient comes forward in the chair until his heels are on the floor, brings his shoulders forwards to the erect position, places his crutches at each side in line with his hips and slowly raises himself, bringing his feet back towards him, then extends his hips by pressing on his crutches, with his shoulders externally rotated to reinforce his back extensors. When his hips are over his feet and he has gained his balance, he brings his crutches forwards and places them on the floor.

2. The patient brings himself forward in the chair, crosses one leg over the other, turns completely round in the chair, supported on the chair arms, hitches his legs forwards one at a time, takes one crutch and hangs it ready on his forearm, puts his hand back on the chair arm, takes the other crutch, extends his hips and stands with that crutch while getting the other into position. This method is less strenuous than the first, but the patient has to be adept at walking backwards to get away from the chair.

Steps. The patient learns to lift himself up on to a step, first placing his crutches up on the step and then lifting his pelvis until his feet can be put on the step and his balance regained by extending his hips.

Coming down, he keeps his crutches up on the step, lifts his pelvis and extends his spine and hips until his feet are over the edge, then lowers until his feet are on the ground, extends his hips and gains his balance, then brings his crutches to the ground.

This practice is essential for getting up to and down from kerbs and into and out of a house with a doorstep.

Stairs. If possible, the patient first attempts climbing stairs which have two strong bannisters. He learns to lift his feet up step by step, in the same manner as above, but if the stair has a 'lip', he must either lift his feet backwards as he goes up, or turn them sideways, to avoid catching them on the edge.

Chair practice. For the majority of patients, their life is going to be spent in a wheelchair, therefore it is essential that the chair should be comfortable, sturdy, the correct size, as light as possible and capable of being folded into a small area, for putting in a car boot, etc. It is also essential that the patient be able to control the chair; he must learn to 'jump' the front castors up on to a kerb or step, manoeuvre in a small space, between furniture and over carpets and rugs. He should practise getting from the chair into a car seat and back and folding it and putting it in the car, once he is in the driver's seat. An invalid car, propelled either by petrol or electric motor, may be issued to the patient, or he may have hand controls fitted to an ordinary car; several quadriplegics now drive their own cars.

SPASM

Spasm, or involuntary muscle contractions which occur due to the un-inhibited action of the spinal cord below the level of the lesion as the control from cerebral influences is lost, is a major problem in the rehabilitation of patients with spinal cord lesions, and is too vast a subject to be covered here satisfactorily.

When giving passive movements, force and brisk movements should not be applied against spasm. Various methods may be used to inhibit spasm, such as a warm bath, elimination of sudden movement or noise, good positioning and relief of any tension in the patient, if possible. The physiotherapist's hands should be warm and the holds used firm but gentle. All movements should be performed smoothly and the patient encouraged to breathe deeply to relax spasm in the abdominal muscles. Ice is of value because, by relaxing spasticity, it prevents the development of contractures which in their turn will lead to greater spasticity.

Clothing should be comfortable, with nothing tight or restricting.

Hydrotherapy. Immersion in warm water, at blood temperature, showers, and swimming are very helpful in reducing spasm, as well as being an excellent medium for exercise.

SPORT

This is an extremely important part of the rehabilitation of a paraplegic and aids mobility, balance, muscle strengthening, co-ordination, posture and builds up the patient's morale as he finds stimulation in competition and self-confidence when he becomes competent.

Archery, swimming, basketball, fencing, table tennis, billiards, bowls, weight-lifting, field events are among those which patients with cord lesions can learn and enjoy, and archery is the one in which they can compete on equal terms with the able-bodied.

OCCUPATION

The patient is assessed during his stay in hospital by the occupational therapist, and if it is impossible for him to return to his former job, he may be sent to a training centre for the disabled to learn a new trade. There should be close co-operation between physiotherapist, occupational therapist and the medical social worker as well as nursing staff.

HOUSING

If at all possible, the patient should return home, where any necessary alterations such as ramps, pulleys, widening doorways and so on may be arranged by the social worker, in conjunction with the local authority, or he may be moved from a flat or house to a bungalow. If this is not possible, he may go to a special hostel, from which he can go to work, or an estate of bungalows designed for those in wheelchairs, or to a home for the disabled. Wherever he goes, the greater his independence at the time he leaves hospital, the fuller and more normal his life will be.

The patient's relatives are taught how to help, where necessary, especially with lifting for a patient with a high lesion and walking for a patient with a low lesion.

CHAPTER 10

Neuritis and Compressive Nerve Lesions

N EURITIS IS AN INFLAMMATION of one or more nerves, characterised by pain, tenderness, altered sensation and muscle weakness. Each spinal or cranial nerve consists of a varying number of nerve fibres bound together by a supporting framework of connective tissue. The fibres of a typical nerve are motor, sensory and sympathetic, they vary in size, the motor being the largest, and the sympathetic the smallest, in diameter.

POLYNEURITIS

Polyneuritis is a disease in which there is degeneration of peripheral nerves. It is characterised by the fact that many nerves are attacked at the same time, the distal end of the nerves being most affected. The condition is symmetrically bilateral. The cause is not always known but in many cases a toxic substance attacks the myelin sheath. This may be a metal such as lead or arsenic, or an organic substance such as carbon monoxide or sulphanilamide. The toxin may be due to infective conditions. For example, polyneuritis occurs in diphtheria, typhoid fever and influenza. It also occurs in some deficiency and metabolic diseases. Thus it is seen in beriberi, chronic alcoholism and deficiency of Vitamin B_{12}. In the commonest type of polyneuritis—acute infective polyneuritis—the cause is uncertain, but it may be due to some organism whose toxin has a special affinity for the lower motor neurones.

Pathology

The pathological changes in polyneuritis closely resemble those of Wallerian degeneration, but are rarely so extensive or complete. The medullary sheath breaks up into fatty droplets; the Schwann cells multiply, some acting as phagocytes; the axons tend to split up but seldom completely disappear. These changes are most severe at the distal part of the nerves, though the whole length may be involved.

As a result of these changes function is impaired. At first pain, deep tenderness and paraesthesia are most outstanding, but, according to the degree of degeneration, there will be sensory loss, diminished reflexes and muscle weakness.

In most cases the onset is insidious, the patient complaining of fatigue and aching in the limbs, a feeling of numbness in the hands and feet, and cramp in the calves of the legs and plantar muscles. On examination, deep tenderness is found and deep reflexes are absent or difficult to obtain. If the condition is allowed to progress cutaneous sensibility becomes increasingly diminished, and in many cases postural sense is lost so that, if the patient can move at all, he is markedly ataxic. Muscular weakness gradually makes its appearance and progresses until the patient is no longer able to get about.

Certain features are more noticeable in one type of neuritis than in others. In lead neuritis the radial nerves are most involved, there are no sensory changes, but the patient suffers from bilateral weakness of the extensor muscles of the wrist and metacarpo-phalangeal joints of the fingers. In alcoholic neuritis degeneration is most marked in small branches of the anterior tibial nerve. Severe cases show numbness and tingling in hands and feet, cramp-like pain in the legs, ataxia, and marked weakness particularly in the dorsiflexors of the ankles. This results in dropping of the feet and a 'high-stepping' gait.

Arsenical neuritis closely resembles the alcoholic type but marked cutaneous hyperaesthesia occurs, and other manifestations of arsenical poisoning, such as skin eruptions, may be found.

Neuritis occurring as a result of diabetes is characterised by pain in the limbs, deep tenderness, and absence of the ankle jerks. In fairly severe cases postural sense is diminished and ataxia is therefore present.

In diphtheritic neuritis, a paralysis appears in the fifth or sixth week after infection and usually involves only one nerve.

Pink disease, like diphtheritic neuritis, occurs in children. In this type of neuritis general symptoms are more marked, the child being irritable, and suffering from lack of appetite, sleeplessness and erythematous rashes. There is hypotonia of muscles, lost tendon jerks and analgesia.

Prognosis. The majority of cases of polyneuritis show complete recovery, provided the toxin can be found and eliminated, and fibrous contactures and deformities have not been allowed to develop. Once the irritant is removed, regeneration of the myelin sheaths and axons will occur. The time of recovery will then depend on the extent of the degeneration.

PRINCIPLES OF TREATMENT BY PHYSIOTHERAPY

The first great essential is rest, in order to prevent over-use of the weakened muscles and because in some patients the heart is attacked by the toxin or the vagi may have been involved. During the period of complete rest steps are taken to find and eliminate the toxin responsible and to build up the patient's general strength and resistive powers. It is also important to deal with the local condition, and this is where the physiotherapist can help. During the period of paralysis or muscular weakness it is essential to maintain the nutrition of the muscles and, in fact, of the whole limb. The prevention of deformities and stiff joints is an important object of treatment. As the muscles begin to recover all possible assistance is given to aid their restoration to normal strength. The physiotherapist will carry out these aims as in any lower motor neurone lesion, but certain special points have to be considered. At the beginning of treatment the limbs may still be tender and the patient unable to tolerate massage or the application of splints. Gentle heat and passive movements may be the only suitable physical measures. Great care is taken to support the limbs by pillows and sandbags and to prevent the pressure of bedclothes by cradles. It must also be remembered that there may be some sensory loss and any form of heat or electrical treatment must be used with caution. Treatment is brief, so that the patient is not tired.

ACUTE INFECTIVE POLYNEURITIS

This is the most common form of polyneuritis in Britain today. It not only attacks the peripheral nerves but also the spinal cord and occasionally the brain. Both inflammatory and degenerative changes are present. Changes occur in the cells of the anterior horns of the cord and in the posterior nerve root ganglia. The meninges are congested. The whole course of the lower motor neurones is affected. The onset is usually sudden, there is a rise of temperature, headache, vomiting, pain in the back and limbs and stiffness of the neck. After a short period there is a sudden onset of paralysis, often beginning in the lower extremities and involving all muscles. It then affects the arms and may spread to the trunk and respiratory muscles. The paralysis is of the lower motor neurone type and accompanied by lost or diminished reflexes and slight muscle wasting. Sensory disturbances are also present. At the onset there will be pain and paraesthesiae and muscles will be tender. Later there will be diminished or lost sensation. Often there is cardiac dilatation and other symptoms of toxaemia.

Though the condition bears some similarity with poliomyelitis it differs in that all muscles are affected and there is sensory involvement.

The prognosis varies according to whether the disease is epidemic or sporadic. In the former case the mortality rate from respiratory paralysis or broncho-pneumonia is high. In the latter recovery usually occurs but it is slow and often not complete.

TREATMENT

There is no specific treatment for this condition but corticosteroids may help. Very careful nursing is needed and the patient may require a respirator.

The patient is often confined to bed for some weeks, usually as long as weakness of the trunk muscles is still present, since any exertion calling for increased respiratory effort might cause respiratory paralysis.

Physiotherapy will be needed to deal with the chest, if the respiratory muscles are involved; to prevent contractures and stiff joints; to aid circulation and re-educate weak and paralysed muscles. It will be carried out on the lines indicated for acute poliomyelitis (see Chap. 7) remembering that sensory changes are also present.

BRACHIAL NEURALGIA

The term neuralgia is chosen in preference to neuritis because it covers a much wider field. The term signifies pain in the region of the brachial plexus or in the distribution of the nerves originating from the plexus, without giving an indication as to the cause, whereas the term neuritis indicates an inflammation. Brachial neuralgia, even better designated as brachialgia (pain in the shoulder region and arm), arises from a great variety of causes. These may be divided into those in which there is local irritation of the nerve roots, brachial plexus, or peripheral nerves and those where the lesion is in soft tissues, the pain being referred.

CAUSES

One or more roots or nerves of the plexus may become inflamed as a result of a neurotrophic virus. This, however, is not common. Very occasionally, following the injection of diphtheria antitoxin or of vaccines, a severe paralytic neuritis develops. These are illustrations of what might be known as a primary neuritis.

More often irritation of the nerves is secondary to some other condition. Certain factors may cause compression or stretching of the nerve and this results in inflammation of the nerve sheath. In the cervical spine, tumours, tuberculosis, osteo-arthrosis and protruded intervertebral discs may all be responsible. In the region of the brachial plexus a group of abnormalities affecting the thoracic outlet may be responsible. In the arm the ulnar or median nerve may be irritated by pressure or, in the case of the ulnar nerve, by stretching resulting from an increasing carrying angle. Pain may be felt in the shoulder or arm from visceral lesions, as, for example, the pain along the medial aspect of the arm in coronary thrombosis and angina. It may also be the result of arthritis of any of the joints of the upper extremity. Lesions in the muscles, ligaments or capsule of the shoulder joint, may be the cause of brachial neuralgia. Further, pain may arise from soft tissues of the elbow, forearm, or hand, though these are less often at fault.

DISTINGUISHING FEATURES

The first essential in treatment is the ability to distinguish between the neuralgia due to irritation of the nerves and that due to involvement of other tissues.

Pain is present in both types of neuralgia. In each it is persistent at rest and on movement, but in the first type it is increased by any movement which stretches or causes compression of the affected nerve root or peripheral nerve. In the second type movements which stretch the plexus do not increase the pain but those which exert traction on the muscle, ligament or capsule which is the cause of the trouble will aggravate it.

The site of the onset of pain may help in deciding the type. If the neuralgia is due to lesions of the nerve root or plexus, pain will usually be felt in the neck first; whereas if it is due to a lesion such as a shoulder joint capsulitis, it will first be felt deep in the shoulder.

If the nerve root is involved, pain is usually of two types: a lancinating pain in the cutaneous distribution of the affected root, and a dull burning pain felt in the deeper tissues supplied by this root. Pain which is due to lesions in other tissues is more in the nature of a dull ache.

Tenderness. Tenderness can often be elicited by squeezing the muscles supplied by the affected nerve. Tenderness may also be felt in the posterior neck muscles in lesions of the vertebral column. If the soft tissues are the source of trouble there will be no tenderness in the course of the nerves, but there will be tenderness at the site of the lesion. Thus, for example, if periarticular fibrositis is the cause of pain in the arm, tenderness will be elicited round the shoulder joint and in the muscles acting upon it.

Paraesthesiae and numbness. Tingling, a feeling of pins and needles, and a complaint of the fingers feeling numb will only be present if the nerve roots or nerves are affected, since these symptoms are due to irritation of sensory nerve fibres. Their presence in brachial neuralgia is almost always indicative of nerve involvement.

Reflexes may be altered in brachial neuralgia due to compression or stretching. If the sixth nerve root is involved the biceps jerk may be diminished; if the seventh root is compressed or stretched the triceps jerk will be weakened. Reflexes will remain unaltered if the lesion is of other tissues.

Muscle weakness may be present in the muscles supplied by the affected root, particularly if there is prolonged stretching or if the nerve is involved in increasing pressure. In severe cases of disc protrusion, for example, marked paresis may develop. Localised muscle weakness does not occur in the second type, though if the condition is acute there may be diffuse muscle weakness arising from disuse.

Herniated cervical disc. A postero-lateral protrusion of a cervical disc tends to protrude into the bony tunnel through which the cervical nerve issues. This tunnel is narrow and is completely filled by the nerve roots, spinal nerve and blood vessels. This additional material, therefore, results in compression of the nerve and veins, with congestion, swelling of the nerve and further compression.

These cases are usually characterised by a history of attacks of pain and stiffness of the neck. Eventually one attack is followed by pain radiating into the arm and made worse by coughing, sneezing and certain movements of the neck, particularly extension because this reduces the size of the intervertebral foramen. Paraesthesiae are felt segmentally and there may also be weakness of the group of muscles whose main nerve supply is from the affected nerve root. Neck movements are usually limited and the neck is often held stiffly and shows a flattening of the normal concavity.

Tenderness may be present over the lower cervical spine and in the muscles supplied by the nerve.

Osteo-arthrosis of the cervical spine. Cervical spondylosis may give rise to brachial neuralgia for several reasons. There may be thinning of the intervertebral disc causing narrowing of the bony tunnel for the nerve, there may be thickening of the capsule of the joint between the articular facets, or changes in the joints of Luschka, or there may be protrusion of an osteophyte into the tunnel. Any of these may cause compression and inflammation of the nerve. The condition is usually insidious in its onset. All movements of the cervical spine may be limited and painful. Pain in the neck may radiate up into the occipital region if the upper part of the cervical spine is involved. X-ray evidence of diminished disc space and osteophyte encroachment on the intervertebral foramen will confirm the diagnosis.

Thoracic outlet abnormalities. Various abnormalities are liable to be present at the base of the neck. These give rise to pain, paraesthesiae, weakness and sometimes circulatory disturbances in the arm, because they cause a stretching or compression of the trunks of the brachial plexus and the subclavian artery. The trunks of the plexus are prone to stretching because, in the erect position, they are angulated as they pass from the neck into the axilla (see Fig. 15). Any factor which increases the angulation may

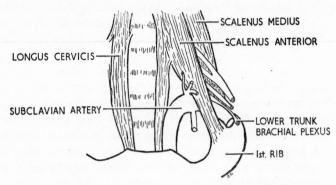

Fig. 15. Diagram to show position of trunks of brachial plexus and subclavian artery in relation to scalenes and first rib.

give rise to symptoms arising from traction. A cervical rib may cause trouble because, if present, the seventh and eighth roots or the lower trunk of the plexus lie on it; their angulation is, therefore, increased and as the rib is lifted on each inspiration there is constant friction. Occasionally there are abnormalities in the insertions of the scalene muscles. If the anterior muscle inserts a little further back or the medius a little further forward, the lower trunk of the plexus and the subclavian artery are lifted up between these muscles and compressed. Scalenus anterior may, for unknown reasons, be in a state of spasm, so elevating the first rib and thus increasing the natural angulation of the neurovascular bundle. If the sternal ends of the first rib and clavicle are unusually high, while the acromial end of the clavicle drops, the subclavian artery and possibly the lower trunk of the plexus may be compressed as they pass between the first rib and the clavicle into the axilla.

Drooping of the shoulder girdle alone may produce stretching and, therefore, symptoms. This drooping may be due either to a decrease in normal tone of the elevators of the shoulder girdle or an incorrect posture in which the postural length of these muscles is too great. Fatigue and unaccustomed heavy use of the arms may contribute towards the first factor.

The syndrome which accompanies these abnormalities is different from either of the preceding cases, since although all the trunks may be affected it is most often the lower trunk which is involved. Pain and paraesthesiae are found, therefore, along the medial side of the forearm, hand and fingers.

If weakness is present it will occur in the small muscles of the hand. Vascular symptoms may also be present. There will then be attacks of coldness, blueness and swelling of the hand, and the radial pulse will be diminished—a sign which is particularly noticed if the arm is dragged down or elevated above the head. In addition there is often aching discomfort at the root of the neck. The syndrome tends to be relieved by raising the arm to shoulder level.

According to the degree of the traction or compression exerted on the neurovascular bundle, so the severity of the symptoms varies. The most intense symptoms are usually produced by the presence of a cervical rib and the least severe by the drooping of the shoulder following fatigue. This latter is probably the cause of the milder syndrome found in the condition known as *acroparaesthesiae*. This occurs most commonly in middle-aged women. There is the sudden onset, usually during the night, of numbness and severe pins and needles in the fingers, sometimes associate with pain. Often it is so distressing that the patient, usually a middle-aged woman, has to get out of bed and rub the hand and swing the arm to get relief. The symptoms quickly subside but may recur during the night. The attack practically always follows a day of hard arm work, the wash day or the day in which much sewing or cleaning has been done.

Ulnar neuritis. The ulnar nerve may be irritated by constant friction if the groove in which it lies at the back of the elbow becomes roughened. It may be subjected to traction if there is an increased carrying angle. In these cases the brachial neuralgia will be limited to the distribution of the ulnar nerve. The pain and paraesthesiae will be felt in the ulnar border of the hand and in the medial one and a half fingers. Muscle weakness may be found in the intrinsic muscles of the hand, excluding the lateral half of the thenar eminence and lateral two lumbricales. It may also be noticeable in the flexor carpi ulnaris and medial half of flexor digitorum profundis.

Median neuritis. The most common causes of this type of brachial neuralgia are bony irregularities round the wrist causing friction of the nerve, or compression of the nerve in the carpal tunnel (carpal tunnel syndrome). These will give rise to symptoms usually limited to the distribution of the nerve in the hand (see Plate XVI). Occasionally, in severe cases of carpal tunnel compression, pain may radiate up the flexor aspect of the forearm to the shoulder.

PRINCIPLES OF TREATMENT BY PHYSIOTHERAPY

Treatment of brachial neuralgia depends entirely on the cause.

Neuralgia due to a herniated disc. If the disc becomes embedded in the body of the vertebra or shifts even slightly, pressure on the nerve root may

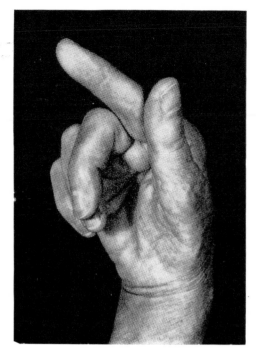

Plate XVI (*see p.* 231)

Median Neuritis

(a) Showing pointing fin-
ger on attempted flexion

(b) Same case. Showing
flattening of thenar eminence

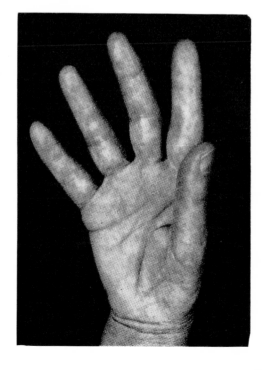

be relieved and inflammation should then subside. This may occur spontaneously with rest, and *rest* is therefore the first measure to be tried. If pain is severe the patient is usually treated in bed, with the head adequately supported on pillows and the arm resting in abduction so that the strain on the inflamed nerve root is avoided. As pain subsides the patient is allowed to get up, wearing a large arm sling, and when pain has completely disappeared strengthening exercises for the neck muscles are begun. Training of the correct posture of the head is important. No treatment for the arm is required unless there is muscle weakness, when exercises will be given. If this treatment proves unsuccessful, head traction may be used; this also will be followed by strengthening and postural exercises. Manipulation of the neck under an anaesthetic is occasionally carried out, and again will be followed by strengthening and postural exercises. In a few cases, especially those in whom pain is unbearable or muscle weakness is marked, a cervical laminectomy may be undertaken. Some surgeons allow free movements of the neck after a period of seven to ten days, others order a plastic or leather collar which may be taken off for toilet purposes and gentle exercises. In either case any weakness of arm muscles will be treated by exercises and if necessary by electrical stimulation.

Whatever the method of treatment adopted by the physician, the exercises aim at getting a good carriage of the head and strong muscles to support the cervical spine, thus lessening the danger of further herniation.

Neuralgia due to cervical spondylosis. In this type also the chief aim is to relieve pain in the arm by reducing the compression of the nerve root and so relieving congestion. Sometimes intermittent traction will result in stretching of the thickened periarticular tissues or cause slight shifting of the contents of the tunnel. This may be carried out either in the ward or in the physiotherapy department by the physiotherapist. Occasionally gentle manipulation of the neck will relieve pain, possibly because it may break down adhesions or free an adherent nerve root. If these measures are not successful a collar may be ordered.

Improvement is sometimes gained by the use of physiotherapy, which may include traction, short-wave therapy, and exercises. Short-wave diathermy is employed in an attempt to soften the thickened periarticular tissues and so to relieve pain and assist stretching. Exercises are used to strengthen the muscles and maintain or increase the range of neck movements. They are particularly valuable to train the patient to hold the head erect. If the head is carried forward the cervical spine is shortened and this may increase compression. As correct a posture of the head as is possible should become a habit. Thus a treatment for brachial neuralgia due to cervical spondylosis might consist of short-wave diathermy, traction, passive movements of the neck, followed by free and resisted active head movements and training in posture.

The arm will only require treatment if there is any muscle weakness or wasting.

Neuralgia due to abnormalities at the thoracic outlet. The first object is to gain a new postural length of the elevators of the shoulder girdle, so that the point of the shoulder is raised and angulation of the neurovascular bundle is relieved. The patient is, therefore, shown the present position of the shoulders, and an explanation is given as to how this position is responsible for her symptoms. She is then taught to take and feel the correct position. Gradually the new position is converted into a habit by constant reminder and by performing simple trunk, head and leg exercises while maintaining the correct position of the shoulder girdle. If there is weakness of the muscles, though often this is not the case, resisted exercises to the elevators of the shoulder girdle should be applied.

If the patient shows intrinsic muscle weakness or circulatory disturbances, physical treatment may be given, but most often these imply some more serious stretching or a compression and surgical treatment is needed to divide the scalenus anterior or remove a cervical rib. If the diagnosis is spasm of scalenus anterior, short-wave diathermy to the neck and training relaxation of the neck and shoulders are both of value. In addition to physical treatment the patient requires advice. Exercises must be practised regularly. Heavy use of the arms should be avoided. Knitting or sewing should not be undertaken for an hour before going to bed. Heavy weights should not be carried and the patient should sleep with a pillow placed behind and below the shoulder so that the shoulder is lifted up and forward. In this way the strain is taken off the neurovascular bundle at the root of the neck.

Neuralgia due to arthritis of the joints of the upper extremity or lesions of muscle, fascia and tendons. Once more treatment is of the cause rather than of the actual symptoms. Arthritis will be treated according to its type and severity (see Chapter 2, Part II). The treatment of soft tissue lesions has already been discussed (see Chapter 5, Part II). The main essential is a very careful examination of the patient to locate the site of the lesion and an equally careful explanation to the patient as to why the shoulder, for example, is being treated when pain is being felt in forearm and hand.

SCIATICA

This is a condition characterized by pain in the buttock and leg. Like brachial neuralgia it may be the result of inflammation secondary to compression or stretching, or it may be due to lesions of other tissues.

CAUSES

A common cause is a herniated lumbar disc. One or more roots of the sciatic nerve may also be compressed as a result of osteo-arthritis or ankylosing spondylitis affecting the lumbar spine (see Fig. 16). Spinal neoplasm or tuberculosis may also have the same effect. Pelvic tumours may cause pressure on the sacral plexus.

Sciatica is also caused by lesions of the soft tissues of the lumbar region or buttock.

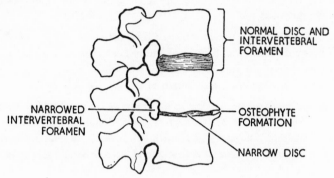

NORMAL DISC AND INTERVERTEBRAL FORAMEN

NARROWED INTERVERTEBRAL FORAMEN

OSTEOPHYTE FORMATION

NARROW DISC

Fig. 16. Diagram to illustrate narrowing of an intervertebral foramen in osteo-arthritis.

DISTINGUISHING FEATURES

Pain is present in all types of sciatica. If the cause is primary inflammation or compression, the pain often extends into the ankle and foot, while if it is a soft tissue lesion it is rarely below the knee. If the nerve root is affected, coughing and sneezing will increase the pain. The pain will also vary in type according to its cause (see page 227). Whatever the cause, straight leg lifting is likely to increase the pain, because this stretches all the soft tissues at the posterior aspect of the hip; but if the foot is dorsiflexed when the leg has been raised to the point of onset of pain, then pain will be increased if the nerve or its roots are inflamed, but not if the lesion is in other tissues.

Tenderness will be found in the region of the lumbar spine if there is compression of the nerve roots, and often in the muscles supplied by the nerve.

Paraesthesiae will only be present if the nerve or nerve roots are irritated.

Reflexes will only be affected if the nerve or its roots are involved. If the first sacral nerve root is compressed the ankle jerk may be diminished or lost.

Muscle weakness may be present in the group of muscles mainly inner-vated by a compressed nerve root. If the cause of compression is a spinal or pelvic neoplasm, muscle weakness usually rapidly progresses to paralysis.

Alterations in posture and gait are liable to occur whatever the cause of the sciatica, but are usually more pronounced if the lesion is one affecting the lumbar spine. Then lumbar scoliosis and sometimes lumbar lordosis may develop.

If it has been decided that the lesion is compression or stretching of one or more nerve roots then it is necessary to examine further to find the cause of the compression.

Osteo-arthritis of the lumbar spine. In this case there has usually been a long history of pain and stiffness of the lumbar region. There is usually limited movement in this area and pain is felt at some point in every movement. There is often also spasm of the lumbar muscles.

Herniated lumbar disc. Herniation occurs more frequently in the lumbar than in the cervical region. In fact this lesion is thought to be the most common cause of lumbago and sciatica. The discs between the fourth and fifth and the fifth lumbar and first sacral vertebrae are the ones most usually affected.

There is often a history of repeated attacks of lumbago, and one attack may then be followed by radiation of pain into the leg. If the fifth lumbar root is compressed, pain may extend from the buttock down the back of the thigh and lateral side of the leg. Involvement of the first sacral nerve root gives rise to pain, which extends from the thigh down the centre of the calf and through the heel into the sole of the foot. Paraesthesiae is often present. In the first case it is usually experienced on the lateral side of the foot, and in the second in the heel and sole (see Fig. 18). Occasionally there is weakness of the peronei and anterior tibial group of muscles. If the first sacral nerve root is compressed the calf muscles may show weakness and wasting and the ankle jerk may be diminished or lost.

On examination tenderness over the lower lumbar spinous processes and lumbar muscles, spasm of sacrospinalis, limited and painful movements (especially in forward flexion), lumbar scoliosis and flattening of the lumbar spine may all be found. Very occasionally symptoms in the leg may occur without accompanying lumbago.

Ankylosing spondylitis. Sciatica is not a common feature of this condition. Once established, ankylosing spondylitis is recognized by the X-ray evidence, the raised sedimentation rate, the stiffness and deformity of the spine and thorax, and the character of the pain, which usually starts rather vaguely in the lumbo-sacral region and tends to spread up the back.

PRINCIPLES OF TREATMENT BY PHYSIOTHERAPY

The principles of treatment depend mainly on the cause.

Sciatica due to osteo-arthrosis and ankylosing spondylitis. This will follow the lines laid down for these conditions (see pages 43 and 75–6). If there is any muscle weakness this will be treated by means of strengthening exercises.

Sciatica due to herniated lumbar disc. The size of a herniated nucleus pulposus usually varies from time to time. This may occur as a result of spinal movements and weight-bearing. In some cases the pressure on the nerve root may be completely relieved. It is because of this possibility that the first treatment tried, if the patient is seen early, is *rest*. Usually the patient is confined to bed for three to six weeks. During this period the strength of the spinal muscles may be maintained by rhythmic contractions of the back and abdominal muscles, and by exercise of latissimus dorsi and trapezius, avoiding movement of the vertebral column. Sometimes the tenderness in the back and leg may be relieved by the use of infra-red irradiation to the back muscles. When the patient begins to get up, exercises to strengthen the spinal muscles, to improve posture, and to gain mobility in the lumbar spine will be given.

One of the most important points in considering the strength of the back is to teach the patient to lift, both from the floor and from above the head, correctly. Trouble in the back often commences following the lifting of a heavy object because so many people lift by extending the back instead of by flexing and extending the hips and knees. No patient should return to his occupation until he can lift correctly.

If rest in bed does not prove successful, traction, manipulation or a plaster jacket may be tried; in either case physiotherapy follows the same lines.

Sometimes none of these means proves successful or if pain is relieved it occurs again later. In some cases the patient may not have reported for treatment until definite muscular weakness or paralysis has developed. In these cases a fenestration operation or laminectomy may be carried out for the removal of the protrusion. The patient is then nursed in the side lying position for the first three to four days being turned two hourly. He can usually lie on his back on the fourth day and get up between the fifth and seventh days.

The time at which physiotherapy treatment may begin depends upon the surgeon. Some surgeons prefer to allow considerable time before any systematic course of exercise is started and a period of two to three weeks may elapse before physical treatment is begun. Others advocate early activity and therefore treatment is begun immediately.

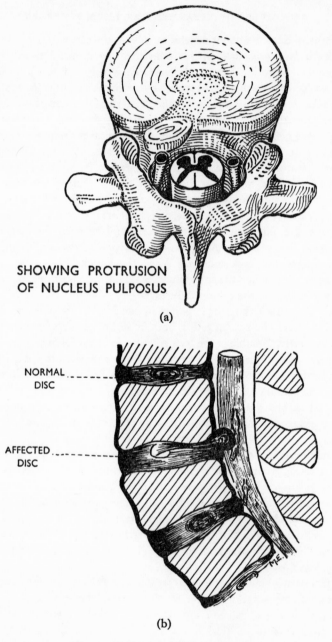

SHOWING PROTRUSION
OF NUCLEUS PULPOSUS

(a)

NORMAL
DISC

AFFECTED
DISC

(b)

Fig. 17. Prolapsed nucleus pulposus.

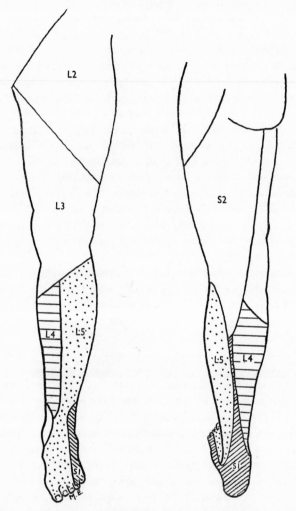

Fig. 18. Cutaneous distribution of L4, L5, S1 nerve roots.

Breathing exercises and coughing, foot and knee exercises are started on the first day and small range hip movements on the second day. Isometric work for the abdominal and back muscles are usually begun between the second and fourth days. Trunk exercises, often in a class, are started about the seventh day when the patient is often allowed to dress and attend the physiotherapy department. These exercises include flexion, rotation and side flexion. The patient is also taught how to bend to pick objects up from the floor, how to sit correctly. When trunk exercises are started, a careful choice of starting positions should be made. Sitting is probably better avoided as it produces most downward compression force on the vertebral column. Lying, prone lying, prone kneeling and standing are suitable as progressive starting positions. The strength of the exercises should be rapidly built up, manual resistance being added as soon as possible.

While strengthening of the back and abdominal muscles is the most important object, it must not be forgotten that faulty posture of the spine and pelvis and limited movement will probably also require attention. The spine will have often been held rigid, in an abnormal posture, by muscle spasm due to pain, for some time before the operation, and this does not right itself immediately after the operation. This is partly because it has become a habit and also because the patient is now afraid to move his trunk in case movement causes pain or damages the sutures. In the course of time, movement will become freer and posture may improve, but the process may be speeded by physical treatment.

Relaxation should be taught in the lying position from the fourth day after operation and this should be progressed, using the sitting and standing positions. The patient should be taught to lie straight and to be able to feel and take up a good posture and this should be progressed to sitting and standing positions.

In many cases, though pain may have been relieved by a laminectomy, muscle weakness and sensory impairment will still be present. These will, in some cases, improve slightly and in others good or full recovery may be expected. In nearly every case there has been a lengthy period before operation has been considered, during which time physical treatment will have been given. If this is so, the exact state of the muscles, in strength and tone, will be known. The physiotherapist will be aware of any sensory loss such as numbness, astereognosis or kinaesthetic impairment. Treatment given before the operation will be continued, modified only by the fact that after the operation the patient may be confined to bed for a few days.

Physiotherapy may therefore be required for the leg muscles as well as for the trunk. The choice of treatment depends on the state of the muscles and may consist of heat to improve the circulation, electrical stimulation to lessen atrophy, passive movements to prevent contractures and deformity, and active exercises to restore power and full function.

When the patient is discharged he is given a lot of exercises, to be practised daily, and instructed to avoid lifting and to rest in the lying position if the back becomes tired.

FACIAL PALSY

Facial palsy is probably due to the fact that the trunk of the nerve is closed for a considerable part of its extent within a bony canal. Oedema of the nerve is therefore likely to result in considerable pressure on the nerve fibres and impairment of their conductivity.

The cause of the palsy is uncertain; cold and exposure may be responsible for inflammatory changes in the muscles and fascia of the neck, with subsequent spread in the sheath of the facial nerve. In this case inflammation may extend along the sheath into the bony canal. Evidence to support this theory rests on the fact that before the onset of paralysis many patients complain of aching and stiffness in the neck muscles, and pain and tenderness in the region of the pinna of the ear and the mastoid process. Since cases seem to crop up in minor epidemic form during the autumn and early winter it is suggested that the condition may be an infective one. Some cases are the result of a geniculate herpes, the inflammation of the geniculate ganglion spreading to the sheath and fibres of the nerve.

Though the condition may occur at any age, it is most common in adults. It is usually unilateral but bilateral affections are seen.

A sudden complete paralysis of all the muscles of expression of one side of the face, with consequent atonia, results in the absence of all expression, the forehead becomes smooth, the nasolabial fold obliterated and the cheek falls away from the teeth and gums. On attempt to close the eye the upper eyelid droops as a result of relaxation of the levator palpebrae superioris, but effective closure is impossible; the eye is therefore inadequately protected and conjunctivitis is a common complication. The lower eyelid sags and tears trickle over on to the face.

Lack of tone in the cheek and muscles of the mouth renders mastication difficult and fluid tends to dribble from the corner of the mouth. In a bilateral case speech is considerably affected. If the nerve is involved before the chorda tympani branch is given off, loss of taste in the anterior two-thirds of the tongue will result.

Recovery depends largely on the extent of the damage to the nerve; if this was sufficient to cause only neurapraxia (conduction block), then a full recovery may be expected within three to six weeks after the onset. In these cases stimulation of the facial nerve trunk behind the angle of the jaw by an intermittent current impulse of 1 mSec. will reveal an equal response on both the normal and the affected sides. If, however, the damage was so severe as to cause degeneration of the axons of the nerve, then no response will be found to stimulation of the nerve trunk.

Where neurapraxia is the cause of the paralysis no treatment is necessary

R

beyond instructing the patient to practise symmetrical facial movements in front of a mirror twice or three times daily. If nerve degeneration has occurred, recovery can take place only by re-growth of the axons from the site of the lesion to the facial muscles. Nerve grows at the rate of one inch per month, and in the case of facial palsy three months is the minimum time before recovery can be expected. During this time the sagging muscles should be supported by holding up the corner of the mouth with an internal dental splint, and the paralysed muscles should be stimulated by interrupted galvanism three to five times weekly. Once improvement begins, the patient should concentrate on practising facial movements, the electrical stimulation being stopped as soon as there is a sufficient voluntary response.

PART V

Principles of Treatment of Diseases of the Skin by using Ultra-Violet Irradiation

BY

TRUDA WAREHAM, M.C.S.P., Dip.T.P.

Principles of Treatment of Diseases of the Skin by using Ultra-Violet Irradiation

ALL PATIENTS WITH SKIN CONDITIONS ARE, in some degree, anxious and worried. The attitude of the physiotherapist can help considerably in the treatment; a serious, moderately optimistic approach is essential. A careful history should be taken and examination made, the treatment must be explained in detail, the reaction that is to be expected and why it is necessary.

At the first attendance a skin test must be done on a comparable area to that which is to be treated; three or four small patches are given different irradiation times and a clear diagram should be given to the patient for him to take home to enter the reactions. If possible he should attend the following day, so that reactions may be checked.

At each attendance accurate records must be made of the reactions obtained from the previous treatment and of the dose given for the current treatment (i.e. the lamp used, the time and distance). If the skin is peeling another dose cannot be given to this area. The patient should understand the reason for this; and he should also be told that certain drugs can sensitise and that he must report to the physiotherapist if the doctor gives him a different medicine or lotion. The same lamp must always be used.

Progression

In order to maintain an erythema each time, the dose must be increased. Using an air-cooled mercury-vapour lamp, it has been stated that the following increases are necessary: E.1. twenty-five per cent; E.2. fifty per cent; E.3. seventy-five per cent. In practice these are usually found to be excessive and considerably less, in each case, will maintain a dose.

When using the Theractin (fluorescent tubes arranged in a tunnel), very small increases only are necessary to maintain an E.1 and, of course, the same lamp should be used each time. Great interest and encouragement forms an integral part of the treatment.

Angle of incidence

Use should always be made of the Cosine Law. It is essential that the rays strike the centre of an area at right angles. On a curved area there will be a diminishing reaction round the edges.

ACNE VULGARIS

This is a chronic inflammatory disease of the sebaceous glands of the face, neck, chest and back.

AETIOLOGY

It occurs mainly at puberty when the sebaceous glands are frequently over-active. There is often a family history. Young men are more affected than young women and it may be associated with such alimentary disorders as constipation.

It is now thought that acne results from a stimulation of the follicles from androgens and that hyperkeratinisation at the mouths of the follicles causes a mechanical obstruction which forms a comedo or blackhead, this stops sebum from escaping. The gland continues to secrete, so cells gradually accumulate, later suppurative changes may follow. As the acute stage subsides, an indolent bluish-red nodule is left and finally a scar. The affected skin is usually greasy and coarse, and has areas of lesions in all stages.

Treatment by Physiotherapy

This aims at causing peeling of the skin at regular intervals and thus to hasten healing of the lesions and therefore to minimise scarring and generally to improve the skin condition.

Preparation

The skin must be clean and recently washed. The face should be washed immediately beforehand.

THE FACE. The hair is held back from the face by clips. Vaseline petroleum jelly is put along the *margin* of the upper lids, and a very narrow piece of wool is held by this along the line of junction of the two eyelids. This must *not* be a large piece of wool covering the upper lid (see Fig.19). The same neck-wear must be worn each time.

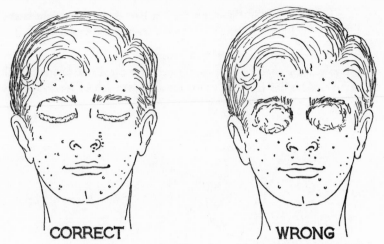

CORRECT WRONG

Fig. 19. Treatment to face by ultra-violet radiation in acne vulgaris.

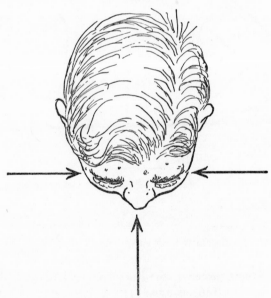

Fig. 20. Treatment to face in three aspects in acne.

Technique I.

An E.2 is given, repeated at about ten to fourteen days to any area, depending on the rate of peeling. The rounded contours of the face and back enable smooth overlap of irradiation aspects without protective towels.

The face is best treated in three aspects, left lateral, anterior, right lateral (see Fig. 20), the burner being at the level of the zygomatic arches.

The back should be treated in four aspects:

(*a*) Two oblique superior aspects, the reflector tilted to lie parallel with the neck-shoulder line (see Fig. 21) If the skin over deltoid is affected, the hands should be placed on the hips.

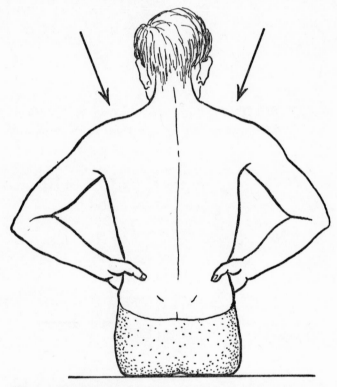

Fig. 21. Treatment to neck shoulder line of the back in acne.

(*b*) Two oblique posterior, the burner being level with the inferior angle of the scapula. Patients usually attend only once a week, so that the face is treated one week, the back another; by the time that the next week comes round, the face will have stopped peeling and be ready for another irradiation.

The mercury-vapour lamp has been found to be more effective than the more restricted spectrum of the fluorescent tube lamps.

Technique II

With this method ultra-violet irradiation is used as a general skin tonic. The patient is instructed to rub his face briskly for a *timed ten minutes* with a new piece of lint and soap and water once a day. This in effect will cause desquamation. This is done at home. The areas are irradiated twice a week with a minimal E.1. Great care must be taken to maintain the dose, and not to let the patient get more than this. For obvious reasons in most cases, this method is only possible for areas that the patient can 'wash' himself, i.e. the face.

ALOPECIA AREATA

This condition is characterised by patches of baldness of the scalp.

AETIOLOGY

Any age may be affected, but mainly young adults. There is often a history of anxiety or strain, some authorities consider that there is an endocrine dysfunction.

Changes

The hair follicles become atrophic, there is a reduction of pigment in the skin and hair bulb. This atrophy starts in the papillae and extends up the hair shaft. Hair ceases to be formed in the affected patches and, in the area immediately surrounding, it tends to break off. The skin becomes atrophic and smooth.

Signs and symptoms

These may appear suddenly or over a period of a few weeks. One or more rounded patches appear which may enlarge, or run together. If the baldness is complete it is termed *alopecia totalis*.

TREATMENT BY PHYSIOTHERAPY

At the first attendance it should be explained that treatment cannot have an obvious effect at once; hair may continue to fall out for about three weeks, and is unlikely to start growing for several weeks after that; so patience and conscientious attendance is essential. A good erythema dose should be given and maintained. An E.3 requires such a quick progression that very long irradiation times soon bring the course of treatment to an end. An E.2 is equally effective, and gives a longer course.

The more irritating rays from a mercury-vapour lamp spectrum have been found to be more effective than those of the fluorescent tube (Theractin).

Stimulation of the skin by high frequency sparks is an extremely useful part of the treatment. It should be given at every attendance for fifteen to twenty minutes, to the whole scalp, fairly strongly, immediately *before* irradiation. This is an added stimulus.

If there are more than two patches of baldness, or with alopecia totalis, two aspects should be irradiated at each attendance. If, when the patient comes for treatment, all areas are peeling, the high frequency can be given for longer. When a course of ultra violet is completed the patient may continue to attend once or twice a week for high frequency, until the next course of ultra violet is started.

Newly grown hair can be felt before it can be seen; this should be shown to the patient and is a great encouragement. An accurate plan of the areas affected must be drawn and each patch clearly described or numbered; this plan must be kept up to date as the patches change.

An alopecia totalis is irradiated from several aspects, sometimes four aspects: Left antero-superior, right antero-superior, left and right postero-superior. Some physiotherapists prefer five: right lateral, left lateral, anterior, posterior and superior.

Technique

The area to be treated is rubbed with industrial spirit to remove grease, surrounding hair is kept back by hair clips and the face is protected with a towel (held firmly by a large spring clip). The tips of the ears may need to be shielded with wool.

The patient should be told that, as new hair grows in, it may be a different colour but it will soon change and match up.

ECZEMA OF THE ELDERLY

This condition benefits very well from generalised irradiation using E.1 doses twice a week and the Theractin lamp where this is available.

PSORIASIS

This is one of the commonest skin diseases. All ages are affected, men more than women, and it is commoner in northern climes. Psoriasis is a chronic inflammatory disease characterised by clearly defined, dry, rounded red patches with silvery scales on the surface.

AETIOLOGY

The cause is unknown, the tendency to it is hereditary. The general health of the patient is usually good. It does appear that the psoriatric skin is better in a sunny climate. A variety of factors may provoke a first attack; friction of the skin, psychological trauma, metabolic upsets, infections or debility, pregnancy or menopause. In some cases it is associated with rheumatoid arthritis.

Symptoms

At first the patches are small but these gradually spread and they may so enlarge that only small areas of skin remain unaffected, the scales become thicker. Some areas are more commonly and more obstinately affected: the backs of the elbows, the fronts of the knees, the sacral region, the chest wall and the scalp. The face is rarely affected. In chronic cases the nails may become involved. In a very severe case the scaling may be so extensive that the floor may be covered with scales when the patient has undressed.

Prognosis

The long term prognosis is not good, but the immediate prognosis for an attack is good, though it tends to recur.

TREATMENT BY PHYSIOTHERAPY

There are a very wide variety of techniques. General irradiation is essential, the best results being obtained from the Theractin. Ultra-violet irradiation is given in conjunction with tar applications. E.1 doses should be given two or three times a week, and in very severe cases daily treatment is indicated. As previously stated, the progression times with the Theractin are very small. An E.1 may be maintained on most patients by increasing by a quarter of a minute until four minutes are reached, then by half minutes to eight minutes, and by three-quarter minutes to twelve minutes and by one minute to fifteen minutes.

The following is one technique:

The patient soaks in a 'tar bath' (two ounces of liquor picis carb.) for ten minutes. This is followed by a brisk towelling and the skin is then lightly rubbed with liquid paraffin. He then lies on his back on the couch, the tunnel is lowered, all clothing is removed.

After irradiation is given to the antero-lateral aspects, he turns onto his face and is given the same dose to the postero-lateral aspects. He then rubs down gently to remove the liquid paraffin. A fairly long course of treatment may be necessary.

If one or two small obstinate patches remain, these may be given localised irradiation E.2 doses.

If only a mercury-vapour lamp is available, the treatment is more complicated. Eight irradiations must be given. At first four at each attendance, two anterior and two posterior one day, and two right lateral and two left lateral the next (see Fig. 22).

Later as the condition improves fewer areas are irradiated at a treatment.

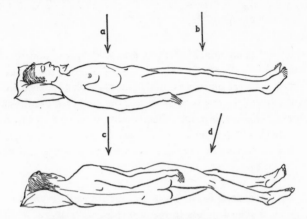

Fig. 22. Treatment of psoriasis by irradiation to the anterior, posterior, right and left lateral aspects.

WOUNDS

The types of wound which benefit most from ultra-violet irradiation are those which are indolent and infected such as gravitational ulcers and pressure sores.

The surrounding skin. A fairly large area of surrounding skin should be given an E.1, and the reaction maintained by correct progression. This should be done each time before irradiating the wound.

The wound. The important maxim here is, 'One cannot overdose an infected wound, but inadequate doses are a waste of time'.

The surrounding skin is carefully masked with yellow Vaseline petroleum jelly and wet cotton wool. This is a quick technique to do and gives a very accurate edge using the non-touch technique. All other areas of skin nearby are then covered with towels. The dose should be at least five times an E.4.

The air-cooled mercury vapour lamp with the beneficial infra-red rays in its spectrum, appears to be more effective than the Kromayer lamp. Ultra-violet irradiation should be given two or three times a week, provided the skin sensation in the surrounding area is normal.

PART VI

Physiotherapy in Paediatrics

BY

BARBARA KENNEDY, M.C.S.P.

Physiotherapy in Paediatrics

THE SUBJECT OF PAEDIATRICS is one requiring many years of study and experience and cannot be condensed into a single chapter. It is only possible to give an idea of the approach and treatment of babies and young children and to describe some of the more common congenital abnormalities.

INTRODUCTION

Watch any child at play. See how often he shifts position; from stretching to squatting, from one leg to hands and knees. By observing and working with children the physiotherapist can learn much from them about themselves. Obviously children enjoy movement, and as a great deal of treatment is based on this fact, the physiotherapist must be aware of the normal motor behaviour of various age levels (Table I). She must also acquire an understanding of the child so that she can help him to help himself.

As children differ from adults in many ways and require a completely different outlook and tempo, it is better if they can be treated in a separate place. The atmosphere should be informal and relaxed, and the children handled calmly and firmly, not rushing or fussing over them, but giving them time to take stock of their surroundings before treatment begins. Much frustration can be avoided by realising that a child cannot be hurried, and cannot reason under the age of five. The best co-operation can be obtained by constant encouragement and liberal praise, for which most children will work really hard. One child varies tremendously from another and treatment must be adapted, not only to their physical and mental level, but to their particular personality. In treating babies and toddlers, use is made of their natural developmental and play activities (Table II). Very small babies will startle and cry at loud noises and sudden movements, and should be approached and handled quietly and with care. Babies move fast and must never be left in any place off which they could roll. They are safe lying on a blanket on the floor. In the wards cot sides must be raised and locked before the physiotherapist leaves.

As the child gets older, use is made of toys, simple apparatus, easy games and imaginative play. As long as the physiotherapist has her objective clearly in mind, she can then adapt the child's activity to achieve this end.

With outpatients, the parents play an important part in treatment and a good relationship between them and the physiotherapist is essential. In many conditions physiotherapy will not succeed without the full co-operation of the mother and everything must be done to encourage her to persevere with treatment at home. At the first visit the physiotherapist must explain the importance of treatment, the expected result, and the length of time it is likely to continue. Time must be spent in listening to the parents' point of view and in arranging the appointments to fit in with the mother's commitments to the rest of her family.

Having acquired all possible data from the medical notes, the mother's account, and her own observation of the child during the interview with the parents, the physiotherapist can decide whether to treat the child herself, afterwards teaching the mother what to do at home; or to start by teaching the mother to treat the child. The first is the method of choice, if mother is inept or frightened of handling her child. In the latter case demonstration by the physiotherapist should be followed immediately by the mother handling the baby under supervision. Older children are often better treated on their own or with other children. When they have learnt what to do, they enjoy demonstrating while the physiotherapist explains to the parents. The second method, of working entirely through the mother is useful for children between one and three years, for ill, miserable children (it helps if there is free visiting on the ward) and for those who attend only occasionally for home programmes.

HOME TREATMENT

This must be simple, clearly explained and where possible, written down, so that it can be checked at each visit and suitable progressions added. Parents must understand that home treatment *must* be done regularly and encouraged to set aside a definite time each day for the purpose. Some alternative exercises should be given so that the child does not become bored.

In the first twelve months of life, the baby progresses from complete helplessness to a fair degree of independence. The new-born baby has only weak reflex movements, his hands are clenched, his body flexed, and his head flops about unless supported. At a year he is mobile, beginning to stand, feed himself and make his wants known. In between, development takes place in a definite order, one stage leading to the next, as the nervous system develops. The ages given below are the average, but a wide range in either direction may be considered normal.

TABLE I

Major Milestones of Development

One month	Alternate reflex kicking. The beginning of head control with slight extension of the head when baby is prone.
Two months	Eyes begin to focus.
Three months	Extends head and spine in prone position. Head less floppy in other positions but still weak. Turns head to look at object.
Six months	Strong back extensors, pushes up onto extended arms in prone position. Uses alternate kicking movement in prone to creep on his tummy. Lifts head in supine position and begins to sit. Can open and close hands, takes toy, plays with own hands. Rolls over from prone to supine. Will soon be able to roll from supine to prone.
Nine months	Crawls, sits alone, pulls himself to standing.
Twelve months	Walks holding on.
Fifteen to eighteen months	Walks alone.
Two to three years	Stands on one leg, jumps.
Four to five years	Hops. It is interesting to note that there is usually a dominant leg on which the child can balance and jump for some months before the second side catches up.

TABLE II

Methods of exercising various muscle groups at different ages. The ages quoted are the earliest at which the exercise should be attempted

Starting position	Exercise	Age
(1)	Light stroking or tickling over muscles stimulates them to contract.	one month
(a) Supine	For abdominals, trunk side flexors, hip flexors, arms, legs and feet.	
(b) Prone	For back extensors, glutei, hamstrings, rhomboids.	
(2) (a) Supine	Head rotation, to look at rattle.	two months
(b) Prone	Rattle should be moved slowly to give time for eyes to focus.	three months

S

TABLE II *continued*

Starting position	Exercise	Age
(3) Supine. Physiotherapist holds one foot in each hand with her thumb along the sole.	Alternate flexion and extension of the legs. When baby feels pressure on his feet he will push against it.	one month
(4) Supine. Physiotherapist's thumb grasped in baby's hand.	(*a*) One arm circling; passive becoming active. (*b*) Alternate arm raising overhead, and to sides. (*c*) Both arms together, overhead then down to tickle tummy. (*d*) Arms stretched sideways, then taken across body (as in hugging self) to tickle opposite side of chest.	one to three months

All these exercises can be used for mobilising the thorax as well as working the shoulder and arm. Exercises (*c*) and (*d*) can be done with breathing, giving slight pressure on the chest on the second movement, or prolonging the tickling to stimulate coughing.

(5) (*a*) Supine	Extension of both legs against resistance, followed by passive flexion giving slight pressure or tickling tummy or chest. (Works back and leg extensors and abdominals.)	three months
(*b*) Supine legs bent, feet resting on bed.	Physiotherapist holds baby's feet with left hand and with her right tweaks or tickles the buttocks causing the baby to lift them off the bed; if he does not do so she puts her hand under him and does the movement for him till he gets the idea.	three months
(6) Prone (*a*) Across physiotherapist's knee or on flat surface.	Encourage head raising and back extension, attracting attention with toy.	three months
(*b*) Prone on bed	Physiotherapist places hands under baby's chest and lets his feet push against her body. As she lifts him up she will extend his head and back.	six months
(*c*) Held as in (*b*)	If then tipped sideways he will try to keep the upper part of his body upright by working his side flexors and rotators (see Plate XVII (A) and (B)).	ten months
(*d*) Physiotherapist sits with baby across her knees, or with his legs between hers.	Baby bends down to floor and then raises himself (with help at first if necessary) to reach up for toy (see Plate XVII (C) and (D)).	eight months

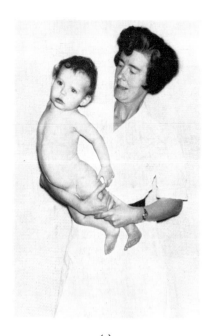

(a)

(b)

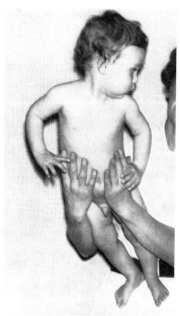

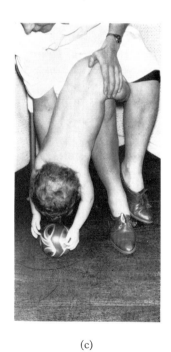

(d)

(c)

PLATES XVII, a, b, c, d.
(see p. 256)

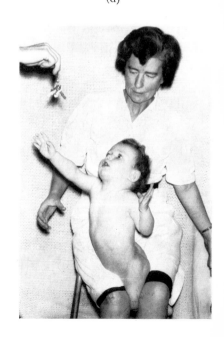

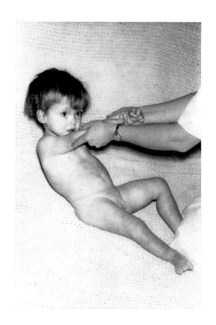

PLATE XVIII

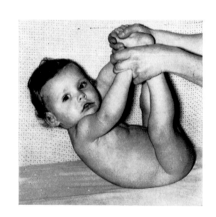

PLATE XIX

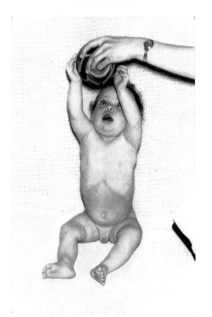

PLATE XX

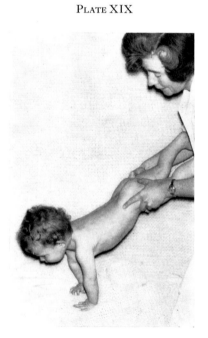

PLATE XXI
(*see p.* 257)

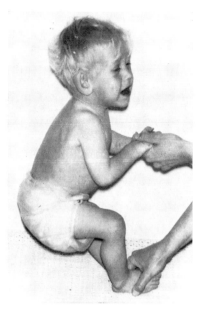

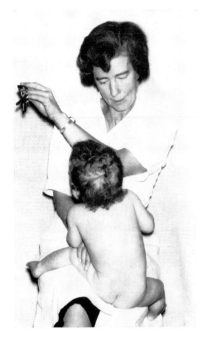

PLATE XXII (*see p.* 257)

PLATE XXIII (*see p.* 257)

VARIOUS EXERCISES

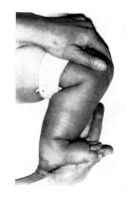

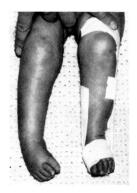

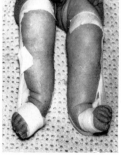

PLATE XXIV
Manipulation in talipes
equino varus
(*see p.* 260)

PLATE XXV
(a)   (b)
Strapping for talipes equino varus (*see p.* 260)

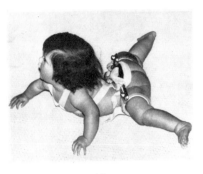

(a)

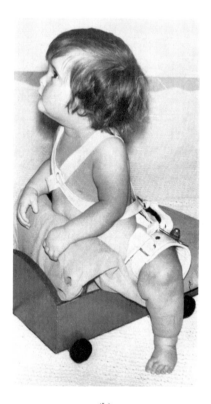

(b)

PLATE XXVI (a) & (b) (*see p.* 263)
Denis Browne Splint maintaining hip abduction but allowing the child to
move the rest of the body freely

TABLE II *continued*

Starting Position	Exercise	Age
(e) Prone on flat surface.	Reach up with one arm for toy supporting himself on the other (trunk rotation).	seven months
(7) Supine, legs bent, feet on bed, arms stretched sideways.	Passive movement of knees from side to side.	three months
	Baby learns to take over.	six months
(8) Supine Physiotherapist holds baby's hands in her right hand. Has her left hand behind his head to give assistance if necessary.	Baby pulls himself to sitting.	four months

Baby's head must not be allowed to loll or to continually hang back. If there is difficulty in lifting the head in supine this may be facilitated by holding the child's elbows and elevating his shoulder girdle (see Plate XVIII).

| (9) Sitting. Child holds own feet in his hands. Physiotherapist has one hand over child's, the other behind his head if required. | Physiotherapist rocks child backwards and then up again. Child takes over (useful for stimulating cough reflex) (see Plate XIX). | six months |

After nine months or so most of these exercises can be continued and progressed, bearing in mind that it is natural for the child to dislike lying still in either prone or supine for longer than a few seconds.

EXERCISES FOR OVER NINE MONTHS

Starting position	Exercise	Age
(10) Sitting on mother's knee or on floor.	Reaching for ball and throwing. Can be adapted for one or both hands and whatever trunk movements are required (see Plate XX).	nine months
(11) Hands on floor, legs held by physiotherapist.	Walking on hands (see Plate XXI).	ten months
(12) Sitting on floor. Physiotherapist holds hands with one hand, feet with her other.	Baby pulls himself to standing (see Plate XXII).	nine months

TABLE II *continued*

Starting position	Exercise	Age
(13) Sitting on mother's knee.	Mother slides one knee down so that baby is tipped sideways. He raises his head and trunk by side flexion (see Plate XXIII).	ten months
(14) Standing (a) alone. (b) Physiotherapist holds knees straight.	Pick up ball from floor (a) Develops balance, extensors of legs and spine (b) Stronger work for back extensors.	eighteen months
(15) (a) Sitting (b) Side sitting	Building bricks, fitting beakers, scribbling, tearing paper—for finger movements and (b) stretching one side of trunk, and balance.	eighteen months to two years
(16) Long sitting	Foot and ankle movements. Knock over bricks by inversion and eversion, make bridge for car by inverting both feet, etc.	two years
(17) Standing. Hands held if necessary.	(a) Stamping, walking on toes. (b) Rock on heels and toes. (c) Stand on one leg—kick ball.	two to three years
(18) Standing (or sitting) at blackboard	Drawing with chalk, for fine finger movements or large shoulder movements.	three years

CONGENITAL ABNORMALITIES

A congenital abnormality is one that is present at birth and therefore was present in the foetus before birth. Very frequently more than one abnormality is present in the same child, for instance a congenital heart condition is often associated with talipes, congenital dislocation of the hips or both. It is normal routine to examine children with one defect for others which may not be immediately apparent.

The three main causes of congenital abnormalities are:

1. Genetic factors.
2. Intra-uterine pressure.
3. Arrested development of the foetus due to an infection of the mother.

The conditions described here are some of those most commonly seen in the physiotherapy department.

TALIPES EQUINO VARUS

As the name suggests, the foot is twisted downwards and inwards. The head of the talus is prominent on the dorsum of the foot, the medial border of which is concave. In severe cases the sole of the foot may face upwards and if untreated the child walks on the dorsum of the foot. The majority of cases are bilateral.

AETIOLOGY

The cause is uncertain but there is often a genetic element. It has been suggested that the development of the foot is arrested before birth, as a result of some unidentified infection of the mother, and that the initial abnormality may be in the bones, with secondary changes in soft tissue. Alternatively, it is possible that moulding of the foot occurs when the foetus lies awkwardly in the uterus and that the primary change is in soft tissue, the bones only becoming misshapen later, if the deformity is not corrected.

There are three components of the deformity:

1. Plantarflexion of the ankle (Equinus). The talus may lie almost vertically instead of in the horizontal position.

2. Inversion at the sub-taloid and mid-tarsal joints. The os calcis faces inwards (Varus).

3. Adduction of the forefoot at the tarso-metatarsal joint. Some cases also have internal rotation of the tibia. There is shortening of tibialis anterior and posterior, and the long and short flexors of the toes. The calf muscles are wasted and the tendo achillis drawn over to the medial side of the heel. Similarly the ligaments and joint capsules on the inner side of the ankle and foot are tight, and the plantar fascia forms a tight thickened band on the medial side of the sole. On the lateral side of the leg, the peronei and lateral ligaments and capsules are overstretched and weak.

TREATMENT

This should be commenced early, on the first day of life if possible, and continued until the child walks. It consists of overcorrection of the deformity, by manipulation, maintained by splinting, and active use of all the leg muscles, particularly the peronei.

Manipulation to obtain overcorrection may be performed on young babies without anaesthesia. In mild cases, where no splinting is necessary, the mother is taught to manipulate the foot each time she changes the nappy. If adequate correction is not obtained in two months, manipulation under anaesthetic possibly with soft tissue releases followed by plaster in full over-correction is necessary. If this fails osteotomy of the os calcis must be considered.

During manipulation the baby's knee is flexed and the lower leg firmly held to prevent any strain on the knee. Each part of the deformity is stretched separately. The manipulations are:

1. To correct the heel.

The heel is pulled down, stretching the tendo achillis, and outwards into eversion. For a good result the heel must be fully corrected in the first two or three weeks of life.

2. To abduct the forefoot.

3. To combine eversion and dorsiflexion taking care that the latter takes place in the ankle joint and not in the sole of the foot. The fully corrected foot can be pushed up and out so that the dorsum of the foot touches the outer side of the leg. (See Plate XXIV.)

Splinting: May be by strapping, Denis Browne splints or plaster of Paris. The splints and plaster will probably be applied by the doctor, and maintain the feet in eversion and dorsiflexion. One inch zinc oxide strapping, following the lines of the manipulations described above, may be applied by the doctor or by the physiotherapist under his direction (see Plate XXV (A) and (B)).

To start with, strapping is renewed every two or three days until full overcorrection can be maintained without undue circulatory disturbance. This is generally in two to three weeks if treatment has been started early. It is then sufficient to renew the strapping weekly or fortnightly. Some form of splinting must be maintained until the child is standing, when its own body-weight acts as a corrective force. Before this time there is a strong tendency for the condition to relapse.

Exercise: Whatever form of splinting is used, the baby is encouraged to kick (against mother's hands, the end of the pram, or when he is old enough, against the floor). This strengthens his muscles and reinforces the correction of the deformity. Each time the strapping is removed, the peronei can be stimulated by stroking over the muscles or along the outer border of the foot. After a few months, full time splintage may be replaced by night boots, leaving the baby free to exercise during his waking hours, and the parents are taught to move the foot through its full range, to stimulate the peronei and encourage the child to stand.

ADVICE TO PARENTS

Parents must understand:

1. The importance of continuous treatment.

2. The danger of the feet relapsing if treatment is stopped too soon.

3. The necessity of keeping splints or strapping dry. This should not be too difficult if the baby wears plastic pants.

4. The importance of inspecting the toes to check the circulation, particularly after splinting has been renewed. The baby should return immediately to hospital if the toes become blue or swollen.

TALIPES CALCANEO-VALGUS

This is much less serious than the equino-varus deformity and tends to recover spontaneously. The baby is born with the foot in a position of eversion and dorsiflexion. All the anterior tibial muscles are shortened together with the ligaments over the front of the ankle.

CAUSE

It is probable that the deformity develops shortly before birth due to the awkward position in which the foetus lies.

TREATMENT

Consists of gentle stretching of the foot into plantar flexion and inversion. The mother is taught to do this several times a day. If the condition is severe or persists, a padded wooden spatula is strapped over the front of the foot and lower leg, to keep the foot in plantar flexion and inversion.

CONGENITAL DISLOCATION OF THE HIP

Congenital dislocation of the hip (C.D.H.) occurs more often in girls than boys and there is a strong familial and geographic distribution.

Cases are found in siblings or in different generations of the family. Children whose mothers had C.D.H. are likely to have the same deformity and should be X-rayed to exclude this, as early as possible.

Dislocation may occur before or at birth, or, in congenital subluxation, not until the child starts to walk. The acetabulum is shallow, its upper rim is deficient and the roof slopes upwards at a greater angle than normal. The neck of the femur may be inclined more forwards than normal, so that the head easily slips upwards and backwards out of the acetabulum; flattening of the femoral head may occur later from pressure against the ilium when the child begins to bear weight, or from avascular necrosis after forceful manipulation has replaced the head of the femur in the acetabulum. Fatty tissue may fill the shallow acetabulum, the capsule of the joint is stretched and may show hour-glass constriction and the adductor muscles become shortened in their abnormal position.

DIAGNOSIS

This may not be made until the child starts to walk, when it will show the typical Trendelenburg gait, if the dislocation is unilateral, or waddling gait, if bilateral. Trendelenburg's sign is positive if, when the child stands on the affected leg, the pelvis drops down on the sound side. Normally the hip abductors of the standing leg contract to keep the pelvis level. They are unable to do this if the upper end of the femur is unstable and does not provide a fixed point from which the abductors can work. Before the child is old enough to stand, the two most important diagnostic signs are shortening of the leg and limitation of abduction of the flexed hip. Often the first indication is the mother's complaint that she has difficulty in separating the baby's legs to apply the nappy. Suspicions may also be aroused by unequal creases in the groin, unequal gluteal creases and lack of movement in one leg compared with the other side. Bilateral C.D.H. is sometimes more difficult to diagnose although there may still be difference of leg length, bilateral tightness of the adductors and broadening of the perineum. Diagnosis is confirmed by X-ray.

The prognosis is very much better if treatment can be commenced before the child starts to walk, so early diagnosis is of the greatest importance. The physiotherapist should be on the alert to notice and refer possible cases whenever she is dealing with babies, particularly those who have a congenital deformity. Talipes and C.D.H. are frequently found to exist in the same patient.

TREATMENT

In young babies simple reduction may be performed without anaesthetic and maintained by a Frejka pillow or Denis Browne splint. If this is not possible, reduction may be obtained:

1. By manipulation under anaesthetic, often preceded by adductor tenotomy, or
2. By traction to both legs with gradually increasing abduction until the legs are at an angle of 180°.

If all attempts at closed reduction fail an open operation will be necessary. The last three procedures are followed by splinting with the hips in 90° flexion, 90° abduction (the frog position) or in any position in which reduction is most stable. Treatment lasts until the head of the femur has been maintained in the acetabulum for at least one year and the acetabular roof has formed satisfactorily. For the last few months plaster may be replaced by a Denis Browne splint. This maintains the hip abduction but allows the child to move the rest of the body freely (see Plate XXVI (A) and (B)). At this stage the child is encouraged to use his legs by sitting astride a truck or tricycle and paddling himself along. He will also learn to walk and climb. In this way, the rotary movement at the hip joint drives the head of the femur into the acetabulum, so stimulating them both to normal shape and growth. Following removal of splinting the child walks on a wide base, but gradually the gait becomes normal without further treatment. Physiotherapy to teach the child to walk on a narrow base is contra-indicated, as strong adduction too early may cause redislocation.

SCOLIOSIS

This is an immense and highly specialised subject which can be reviewed only briefly here. The deformity is of lateral flexion of the spine accompanied by rotation. It may vary in extent and location, the commonest site being the dorso-lumbar region. Compensatory curves may form above and below the primary one. Corresponding rotation takes place in the rib cage which may later seriously impede respiratory function.

Very severe cases may develop neurological signs due to pressure on nerve roots leaving the spine.

Two types of scoliosis are seen in babies:

1. *Structural Scoliosis*, resulting from the maldevelopment of one or more vertebrae (producing hemivertebrae). The ribs may also be malformed, and may be more or fewer in number than normal. There is adaptive shortening of muscles and connective tissue. Sometimes the deformity increases with growth, but although no improvement can be expected, the condition often remains static and symptom free if there are good compensatory curves.

2. *Idiopathic Infantile Scoliosis* may not appear until the baby is a few months old. Some cases effect a spontaneous recovery in about a year, others progress to severe deformity despite all forms of treatment. Nothing is known of the cause. Changes occur both in bony and soft tissue as the condition advances.

TREATMENT

This is by corrective and supportive splints. If, in spite of these, the curve increases, spinal fusion or other operative procedures must be considered.

PHYSIOTHERAPY

The child may benefit from bilateral exercises for back extensor and abdominal muscles, aimed at improving the general musculature which is often poor. The physiotherapist has an important part to play in obtaining maximum mobility of the thorax and increasing vital capacity. Care must be taken to avoid fatigue.

SPINA BIFIDA

There are two types: spina bifida occulta and spina bifida manifesta. In both types there is a maldevelopment of the posterior arch of one or more vertebrae. The laminae, which may be rudimentary, do not fuse, and the spinous process is missing.

Spina bifida occulta is common and, as it seldom produces symptoms, is frequently diagnosed when the spine is X-rayed for some other condition. Usually the defect is limited to one or two vertebrae, L. 4 and 5 being the most common. The lesion may be marked superficially by a deep dimple, or growth of hair. Occasionally spina bifida occulta is associated with pes cavus.

Spina bifida manifesta implies gross abnormality, both of the vertebrae and the spinal cord. The posterior parts of many vertebrae may be missing between the mid-dorsal region and lumbo-sacral junction. A tumour, consisting of meninges and spinal cord or cauda equina, protrudes through the gap.

A meningocoele is a tumour containing only meninges and cerebrospinal fluid, covered by fatty and subcutaneous tissue and skin. As no nerve tissue is involved, there is no paralysis and the prognosis is good, if the tumour can be removed.

Meningomyelocoele is unfortunately the more common of the two. The tumour is formed by actual nerve tissue covered only by the meninges and epithelium. Life is threatened by meningitis, which may follow infection of the tumour, or by hydrocephalus which may be present at birth, or develop because of an associated malformation of the brain. There is double incontinence, and ascending urinary infections are another hazard. Involvement of nerve tissue results in the destruction of the motor and sensory pathways to the lower limbs. Deformities are often present which may be congenital, i.e. due to maldevelopment, or paralytic, caused in utero by the unequal pull of muscles.

In the past, most of these children died, but with advances in surgery and chemotherapy, an increasing number survive and will be seen more and more in physiotherapy departments and special units.

TREATMENT

Operation to remove surplus tissue, returning nerve tissue to the vertebral canal and repairing the deficiency of skin and fascia, may be performed, preferably within a few hours of birth. If there is hydrocephalus, a Spitz-Holter valve is inserted into the jugular vein to drain excess fluid from the lateral ventricle of the brain. The deformities may be treated on the lines already indicated. Paralytic deformities combined with sensory and vascular disturbances may be considered a contra-indication to forceful manipulation and splinting, which might cause further trauma to the bones or ulceration of the skin. The deformities are then corrected surgically at a few months of age.

The most common deformities are talipes equino varus, hyper-extended knees with limited flexion and C.D.H. Dislocation of the hip is common in the first five or six years, due to the adductor and ilio-psoas muscles pulling against the paralysed glutei and abductors.

Adductor tenotomy is often necessary before the dislocation can be reduced. A few months after reduction, a second operation may be performed to transplant the ilio-psoas posteriorly, so that it functions as a hip extensor and prevents re-dislocation.

PHYSIOTHERAPY

This is important at all stages. Early treatment of the deformities will depend on the doctor in charge. If stretching is ordered this should be done with great care. In all cases the existing range of movement must be preserved or increased. Passive movements of all joints should be performed daily through the maximum possible range. If any active movement is present the baby is encouraged to join in. Alternate flexion and extension of the legs should be performed slowly and deliberately, giving pressure against the soles of the feet to try to stimulate normal kicking. Abduction of the hips should also be particularly encouraged. As he has no superficial or proprioceptive sensation, the child should constantly be shown his lower limbs during treatment. When he is old enough a mirror is useful for this purpose. These children generally have normal musculature above the site of the lesion, and it is important that they should develop the upper part of the body in the normal way. Trunk and arm exercises should be started early, so that the child is strong enough to support himself on crutches by the time he is ready to learn to walk. The baby should be encouraged to lie on his tummy, roll over and sit up at the normal times. Between six and eight months he should start to push up on to extended arms from prone and is encouraged to reach for a toy with one hand while supporting himself on the other. 'Wheelbarrows' (see Plate XXI) and other similar games may be devised to strengthen the arms. Later still, in long sitting, he may be taught to lift himself on his arms, using a block under each hand to make it easier, or if his arms are too short to reach the ground.

Muscle re-education is important after the psoas transplant operation. Hip extension is necessary before a child can be taught to stand and walk, which is at about two years provided the general condition permits. Balance and falling are practised in kneeling and standing before progressing to walking training. Most children require full length calipers with pelvic bands, though some less affected need only below knee appliances. It is essential that all appliances should fit perfectly—always. It is the responsibility of the parents and the physiotherapist to keep a continual watch on the skin condition and on the child's growth, and to see that any necessary adjustments are made immediately. Once a pressure sore has developed it may keep the child off its feet for weeks. Parallel bars or various walking aids may be used in teaching the child to walk, progressing to crutches or sticks. The ultimate aim of treatment is independence which includes not only the ability to be mobile, but the various aspects of self care.

TORTICOLLIS

Wry neck or torticollis is a condition quite frequently seen by the physiotherapist. The child holds its head tilted to the side so that the ear is drawn towards the shoulder on the tight side. At the same time the face looks to the opposite side.

STRUCTURAL TORTICOLLIS

A cervical hemivertebra may be the cause of torticollis, but this is very rare and there is no treatment.

FOETAL TORTICOLLIS

The head is held to one side. The ear on this side is often crumpled and there is moulding of the face and head. The torticollis frequently rights itself in a few weeks without any treatment. The moulding disappears more slowly in about one year.

INFANTILE TORTICOLLIS

This is the type most commonly seen by the physiotherapist.

It is often associated with a sterno-mastoid tumour. A small, hard lump, consisting of fibrous scar tissue can be felt in the muscle belly at birth or shortly afterwards. The scar tissue contracts, so shortening the muscle, the clavicular head may stand out in a tight band, and the head is pulled over into the typical position. The cause is unknown. A fibrous tumour may be present before birth, or a haematoma may result from a traction injury during birth. Facial asymmetry and moulding of the head is often a factor, but this slowly improves as the head is held straight. In untreated cases facial asymmetry may persist and after some years it becomes irreversible.

OCULAR TORTICOLLIS

Occasionally the head is held in the torticollis position without the presence of a tumour or tightness of the sternomastoid. There is full range passive movement, and active correction if the baby is co-operative, but the head always returns to the same position afterwards. In these cases weakness of one eye is the cause and they should be referred to the eye department. Once this is corrected the head is held straight without any further treatment. In older children harm may be done by teaching them to hold their heads straight, if the eye has not been attended to first.

TREATMENT

Physiotherapy consisting of stretching, active exercises and general management, should be started early and is usually successful up to the age of six months. After this time the muscle is more difficult to stretch and although it is worth while continuing with physiotherapy, tenotomy of the sterno-mastoid may have to be considered at a later date.

Treatment must be carried out conscientiously at home, so teaching the parents is most important. It is useful to have a typed or printed list of instructions which the mother can take home and use for reference and to show the rest of the family. These must be very simple, and must be carefully explained and demonstrated by the physiotherapist before she gives them to the mother.

Stretching

The movements performed in stretching the sterno-mastoid are:

1. Side flexion of the head and neck away from the tight side.
2. Rotation of the head so that the face is turned towards the tight side.
3. Both these movements combined, side flexion first, followed by rotation.

Active exercise

At about three months when the baby begins to focus, a brightly coloured rattle is introduced into his line of vision as he lies on his back. It is held about eighteen inches away, and he is given time to fix his eyes on it, before it is very slowly moved round towards the tight side. Each time he 'loses' it a fresh start must be made, until eventually, he turns his head through the complete range.

PART VII

The Management of Physical Disability

BY

MARGARET A. STEWART, F.C.S.P., Dip.T.P.

The Management of Physical Disability

PHYSICAL HANDICAP MAY INTERFERE with the performance of personal activities of daily living or with the adult's ability to run a home or earn a livelihood. In addition, the normal educational progress of the disabled child or young adult may be hindered, and patients of all ages may meet with difficulties in taking part in usual recreational activities or sport.

The aim of a rehabilitation programme should be to gain as much capability and freedom in these spheres as is compatible with the individual's age and condition: it is most effectively fulfilled when all members of the rehabilitation services, and the patient, work together to achieve a realistic goal.

From the physiotherapist's point of view any purposeful treatment which relieves a symptom inhibiting activity or removes any impediment to function is part of rehabilitation. A careful, detailed examination and assessment, both of the patient's motivation and the physical condition, must therefore precede the planning and carrying out of treatment. Suitable therapeutic measures should then be taken to remove those factors which interfere with function and will respond to treatment. Where disability is intractable, independence must be restored by other means such as the provision of personal aids, home adaptations or the services of the Health or Welfare Departments of the local authority. These forms of assistance may be expedient during a long period of treatment to tide over physical difficulty or be permanently provided for the patient whose established residual disability interferes with function.

In a wider field special educational facilities are provided by the State for the physically handicapped child; there are rehabilitation and vocational training schemes for the disabled adult and special arrangements for ensuring the re-employment or resettlement of the would-be worker. Where disability and social difficulties make institutional care inevitable accommodation is available in residential homes, in hospitals for the chronic sick, or in special units run by voluntary organisations.

INDEPENDENCE IN THE ACTIVITIES OF DAILY LIVING

At whatever stage the patient is referred for treatment a careful assessment must be made of functional capability.

The accompanying lists give the basic activities used by the patient in achieving personal independence, and cover four areas of activity:

1. The essential needs of the patient who will ultimately be ambulant, with or without walking aids.

2. The activities and transferring abilities required by the user of a wheelchair.

3. Dressing problems and personal care.

4. Activities of toilet and hygiene.

It is essential, always, to see the performance of an activity and not to accept verbal assurance that it can be done, as otherwise a dangerous performance, or one extravagant of energy, may be overlooked.

Grading may be as follows:

☑ Competent performance
Ⓗ Needs help
☐ Impossible

The standard reached should be recorded in different columns at the first and last attendances: it is helpful, too, to record the date on which a competent performance is achieved, when this has not been possible at the first attendance.

Although the method of performance varies from individual to individual, certain movement components may be essential to the normal carrying out of any one common activity. It is possible, from a knowledge of these, to determine by careful examination what lack or deviation is interfering with the patient's capability and so affecting independence. The physical demands made upon the patient at any one assessment session must be governed by the condition, but it is recommended that the therapist works systematically through the basic activities, so that none is inadvertently omitted.

As the patient needs, wherever possible, to be independent in the home it is essential that assessment and training is carried out on ordinary house furniture and fittings. There should, therefore, be available a divan-type of bed, different kinds of chairs with and without arms, toilet facilities and a bath. In addition, simple aids to dressing, feeding and toilet should be at hand. Elaborate equipment is not essential, but furniture should be capable of variation in height to accommodate the considerable range in patients' requirements. Where there is need to climb stairs practice should

TABLE I
The essential needs of the patient who will ultimately be ambulant

Mobility		First Attend- ance	Date Achieved	Last Attend- ance	Comments
Bed:	Lift hips				
	Roll (a) Right (b) Left				
	Move, all directions				
	Sit erect from lying, and return				
	Maintain sitting balance				
	Sit over bed edge from lying				
	Move along bed edge				
	Stand from bed (height ...)				
Chair:	Sitting balance				
	Lift hips				
	Stand. Chair with arms (height ...)				
	Chair without arms (height ...)				
Standing	With aids				
Balance	Without aids				
	Performance of other activities				
Gait:	Aids used =				
	Walking forwards				
	(a) Backwards (b) Sideways				
	(c) Turn round (d) Carry things				
Steps:	Single (height ...)				
Stairs:	Hand rails (a) Two (b) One				
	No handrails				
	Management of aids				
	Outdoor Activity				
Gait:	Uneven ground				
	Slopes				
	Crossing road. Traffic				
Transport:	Car—driver				
	Car—passenger				
	Bus				

TABLE II
The activities and transferring abilities required by the user of a wheelchair

		First Attend- ance	Date Achieved	Last Attend- ance	Comments
Management:	Propel chair				
	Lock and unlock				
	Lift foot pedals				
	Lift hips				
	Pick up object from floor				
	Stand				
Indoor Transfers:	To/from bed				
	To/from toilet				
	To/from chair				
	To/from bath, shower				
Outdoors:	Rough ground				
	Slopes				
	Step, kerb (Height ...)				
	To/from car				
	Chair in and out of car				
Special Problems:	(Work, kitchen, etc.)				
Home Situation:					
Chair Details:	(Model, modifications)				

be given in the department under conditions resembling those at home, bearing in mind, again, the great variations that are possible in depth and tread of stairs, twists and turns in the flight, the existence or not of carpets, and the availability of handrails.

T*

The problems encountered will differ from patient to patient according to disability and the home circumstances so the help that each requires will vary. For example, the inability to rise to standing from sitting may be overcome by raising the height of the bed, chair or lavatory or the supply of suitably-sited grab rails. A second handrail on the stairs may make it

TABLE III

Dressing problems and personal care

		First Attend- ance	Date Achieved	Last Attend- ance	Comments
Dressing or Undressing:	Shoes				
	Fasten shoes				
	Stockings/socks				
	Fasten suspenders				
	Pants, brassiere, corsets				
	Trousers/Skirt				
	Button garment				
	Zip				
	Slip-over garment				
Hair:	Brush/Comb				
	Shave/Make up				
Feeding:	Grip Implement				
	Transfer food to mouth				

TABLE IV

Activities of toilet and hygiene

		First Attend- ance	Date Achieved	Last Attend- ance	Comments
Lavatory:	On (height...				
	Off (height...)				
	Toilet management				
Washing:	Sponge bath				
	Wash extremities/neck				
Bath or Shower:	In with aids				
	In without aids				
	Out with aids				
	Out without aids				
	Turn taps				

possible for a patient to ascend or descend safely when this would otherwise be impossible, and a ramp, suitably placed, may enable the wheelchair-user to circumvent a step and so get round the house. Dressing or feeding aids may be needed to supplement personal independence when there is disability or deformity of the upper limbs, such as may be shown by the patient with gross rheumatoid arthritis, and special seats may make it possible to get in and out of the bath. It is important that each specific disability is countered by a specific aid, effective in its purpose, and that arrangements for its supply are completed by the time the patient is discharged from hospital.

HOME VISITS

Some points to look for when making a visit to the home

Bed	—Access
	Mattress
	Springs
	Width
	Height
Chairs	—Height of seat
	Type—with arms
	without arms
Lavatory	—Height
	Distance from either wall, basin or bath
	Distance behind
Bath	—Outside height to floor
	Midway width inside
	Total width, outside edge to outside edge
	Distance between bath and lavatory
Doorways	—*Width (where necessary)
Passages	—*Width
	Angle of corners
Kitchen	—General layout
	Height of sink
	Height of cooker
	Height of table
	*Clearance under sink
	*Clearance under table
Outdoor	—Number
Steps	Height
	Tread
	*Available length for ramp
	Possible sites for rails
Indoor	—Number
Steps	Height
	Tread
	Detail of turns
	Floor covering
	Banisters
General layout in home	— All relevant distances
Garden	—Steps
	Slopes
	Type of ground

Essential measurements for Wheelchairs.

When sufficient detailed information about the home is not available from the patient, relatives or domiciliary services, a visit to the home by the therapist who treats the patient and knows the capabilities may be necessary: this may be the hospital physiotherapist, occupational therapist or medical social worker, either singly, or jointly where their combined knowledge may be helpful, or in conjunction with the officer concerned from the local welfare authority. The list on p. 275 may serve as a guide to physiotherapists making a home visit.

Methods of obtaining adaptations

Wherever possible the patient's family or friends should provide aids or make necessary alterations, or arrange that they are done by private contract. In some areas voluntary organisations will help with simple adaptations in the home, and in certain situations occupational therapy departments may undertake the work. This last is of particular value when dealing with the more severely disabled patient, where continuing consultation between all concerned can more effectively solve problems of complex disability, or the timely provision of aids maybring about speedier discharge from hospital. In general, however, the approach for help should be made to the welfare services department of the local authority which has been given powers under the National Assistance Act to provide welfare services and to prepare schemes to help the disabled in their homes. The department is thus enabled to undertake the adaptations for those patients who are 'substantially and permanently handicapped' but it must be noted that there is considerable variation throughout the country in the extent of available services and the agency by which they can be provided.

When a public authority undertakes major home adaptations there must necessarily be a careful assessment of means and scrutiny of estimates which may result in some delay before plans are implemented. The patient or family are expected to cover the cost of any work done or to make whatever contribution is possible: sometimes, if income is small, no charge at all may be made to the patient. Some voluntary societies may give help to patients with particular disabilities, for example, the National Spastics Society, the Muscular Dystrophy Group or the British Poliomyelitis Fellowship. In hospital the social worker undertakes the assessment of the patient's financial means and makes arrangements, if necessary, to raise money from such statutory or voluntary services as are available. In all other situations applications for assistance may be made to the Welfare Officer of the local authority concerned.

Some equipment for the disabled, such as commodes, bed-pans, bottles may be loaned to the patient by organisations such as the British Red Cross Society, and sick-room equipment may also be obtained from the public health department of the local authority. In addition, many aids are now manufactured commercially by private firms or government-sponsored agencies.

Wheelchairs are available under the National Health Service for physically handicapped patients and war-pensioners, and are supplied to the prescription of a hospital consultant. A careful choice should be made of the type and modification that will meet the specific needs and transferring abilities of the individual patient, and the physiotherapist has a very valuable role to play in this aspect of the patient's assessment. Single-seater motor or electrically-propelled tricycles are available for patients whose disability is equivalent to the total loss of the use of the legs: they can also be obtained by the patient with a job whose physical handicap is so severe that without a tricycle the journey to work would be impossible. In suitable cases, disabled war-pensioners who are employable are entitled to the use of Ministry of Health cars on loan.

Despite all efforts some patients may be unable to regain total independence and may need help from relatives, where these are available, or from some of the domiciliary services.

Relatives can play a most important part in helping to achieve successful rehabilitation and should be given guidance in their handling of the patient. Sympathetic relatives should understand that a patient should be allowed to be as independent as possible, and that self-reliance as taught in hospital should be encouraged. Over-protection may be just as harmful as lack of help and understanding, and the patient must be made, wherever possible, to feel a useful member of the household. In appropriate cases, relatives and friends should be taught to give such physical help as is necessary in ways that safeguard themselves and the patient.

Assistance can also be provided from the domiciliary services and may include help with the housework or shopping from the Home Help Service or the provision of meals from the Meals-on-Wheels Organisation. The Home Nursing and Health Visiting Services give valuable help in providing necessary nursing care or in general supervision of the welfare of patients. All these, and other supporting services, may enable the heavily disabled patient to continue living at home when otherwise institutional care might be required.

INSTITUTIONAL CARE

In some cases the patient is unable to return home despite prolonged physical re-training and exhaustive effort to solve social problems. Institutional care must then be provided, and accommodation appropriate to the physical and mental capability may be found in residential homes of the Part III type (so-called because such accommodation became available under Part III of the National Assistance Act). This may be in newer, smaller homes where each resident can live as an individual or in older, larger homes where conditions may be far from desirable. When patients require nursing care accommodation may be found in hospitals for the chronic sick or in special homes run by voluntary organisations with the co-operation of Regional Hospital Boards. It is important that the patient achieves maximal independence before discharge from hospital, for this will decide the type of accommodation allocated and so greatly influence the future way of life.

Co-operation

Team work is essential in the effective rehabilitation of patients with complex disability. Throughout the treatment programme the doctor must direct the efforts of the team and give guidance as to the aspects of treatment to be emphasised, the optimum duration and intensity of the patient's schedule and the realism of the target of achievement. Hospital nursing staff play a large part in the encouragement of independence in the ward, and may, in their turn, require guidance as to the patient's fitness to return home. Members of the home nursing services may supervise the patient's after-care and, particularly in districts where physiotherapy is not available, give such simple rehabilitation care as will prevent physical deterioration or crippling deformity.

The physiotherapist works closely with occupational therapist colleagues in retaining the patient's independence in activities of daily living: the main physiotherapeutic role lies in helping the patient with activities that involve general mobility such as the movements in bed, rising from sitting and vice-versa, walking, stair climbing and transfers to and from a wheelchair. The physiotherapist must, in addition, be able to deal with simple problems of dressing, feeding and toilet but more complex difficulties of this kind may be referred to occupational therapists. Occupational therapists play a particularly valuable role in the retraining of the disabled housewife and in other forms of work assessment.

SPORT AND RECREATIONAL ACTIVITIES

Sport and games of all kinds can play an important part in the rehabilitation of hospital patients and in their subsequent integration within the community. Sporting activities strengthen body musculature, improve balance and promote co-ordination in action; in addition, they provide a strong psychological stimulus, particularly for young people. The physical effect will vary with the sport selected and this, in its turn, must be governed by the nature of the disability; for example, the value of sport in the rehabilitation of the paraplegic patient is now well-known and archery, wheelchair basketball, swimming, as well as field events, are sports in which these disabled patients can participate effectively. Pony riding, too, is an activity in which more and more disabled children can take part. Indoor sports, table tennis, skittles, snooker or billiards can be competitive and can as well be a very valuable means whereby comradeship in the social life of the community is re-established.

The British Sports Association for the Disabled was founded in Britain in 1961 and co-ordinates the activities of many organisations. Its activities enable patients to continue with sport locally after discharge from hospital.

Patients in age groups unsuited to sport, or those who are mentally or physically unable to take part in these more vigorous activities, may also wish to share in different forms of recreation. Local authorities, in some instances, encourage voluntary associations to use social clubs, and transport, accommodation and financial assistance may be provided. Day centres, besides catering for the needs of the disabled and elderly patient, often provide a much needed respite, one day a week or more, for the patient's relatives at home.

EDUCATION

It is the duty of local education authorities to find out which children in their area require special educational help and to provide appropriate facilities. Education may be provided within special schools admitting only handicapped children or arrangements may be made for entry to ordinary schools for those children whose physical disability is not serious. Some children, too handicapped to attend a special school, may be taught at home and sometimes a school may be set up within a hospital where there are enough children requiring teaching to make the scheme practicable. In addition to the schools provided by local education authorities there are a number of schools organised by voluntary societies: in all cases the full cost of the education is met by the local authority, and no contribution is required from the child's parents.

In cities and towns day schools are provided where there are enough physically disabled children living within the area to form a satisfactory working unit. Free transport is provided to take the children to and from school where necessary. In rural areas, or where the children are too handicapped to make daily journeys, boarding school education is provided. Throughout school life the general health of the child is regularly supervised. Any treatment such as physiotherapy or speech therapy is arranged.

As far as their disability allows, handicapped children are given the education for which their intelligence calls, and they can sit for the same examinations as normal children. However, the school leaving age is sixteen years or perhaps older when work is being done for a special examination. Facilities are available for further education and training for those who can profit by them, and local authorities may maintain students in training establishments which have been provided by voluntary bodies. Special arrangements can be made through the Ministry of Labour's Youth Employment Services to find jobs for the disabled school leaver up to the age of eighteen years.

INDUSTRIAL REHABILITATION AND RE-TRAINING

The Disabled Persons (Employment) Act aims to help those who wish to work for a living but are handicapped by disability in getting and keeping suitable employment. Experience has shown that most disabled people can take their place in the working community and hold their own in competition with others if the job is carefully chosen.

At each employment exchange there is a Disablement Resettlement Officer (the 'D.R.O.') who is in touch with local employers and who knows what openings exist for the disabled person in the area. When work has been obtained follow-up action should ensure that the job is satisfactory. The transfer of responsibility from medical to industrial care should begin before medical treatment comes to an end: the D.R.O. should receive an informative report about the patient's condition and capability from the family doctor, the hospital or the Regional Medical Services of the Ministry of Health, and close liaison between those concerned smooths the transfer process: in this connection resettlement clinics can be very helpful.

The Disabled Persons' Register is a voluntary register kept by the Ministry of Labour of persons who are substantially handicapped in obtaining ordinary employment. The advantages of belonging to this register are, for example, that every employer with twenty or more workers has to employ 3 per cent of registered disabled people, and some occupations such as car park or lift attendant are reserved for persons in this category. In addition, employment in most sheltered workshops is restricted to people on the register.

Industrial rehabilitation units comprising various types of workshop, gardens or gymnasia have been established to help persons over the age of sixteen years who have been out of work for some time. In these units they are helped to become accustomed gradually to working conditions and to make themselves fit to do a full day's work. Industrial rehabilitation units are of value in assessing the fitness of the person concerned to go back to former employment or in deciding what kind of job would be suitable in the light of the particular disability. Training for a trade is not given in such a unit but, where it is considered necessary, the patient may be referred to a government training centre for vocational training. The types of training available can range from agriculture to hairdressing and from all kinds of engineering and repair work to commercial subjects. Courses may be residential or non-residential and usually last for a period of six months. Towards the end of this period work is done under actual trade conditions, and on the completion of the course help is given with finding a job. During both these schemes the patient is paid a maintenance allowance according to individual financial circumstances.

Some sheltered workshops, organised either by the Ministry of Labour or voluntary organisations, employ severely disabled men and women who are unable to find employment in other ways. Candidates must be still capable of productive work and be willing to work to the best of their ability.

Home Employment schemes are desirable but their scope and availability at the time of writing are very limited.

CONCLUSION

In a total rehabilitation programme the physiotherapist has an important part to play in co-operation with other members of the team. In order that the patient should benefit most fully from treatment the physiotherapist should understand the role of colleagues and have a comprehensive knowledge of the services that are available to help the patient.

Bibliography

PATHOLOGY

Pathology by J. Henry Dible and Thomas B. Davie (Churchill).
An Introduction to Pathology by G. Payling Wright (Longmans Green).
General Pathology by J. B. Walter, T.D., M.D., M.R.C.P., M.C.PATH. and
    M. S. Israel, M.B., M.R.C.P., D.C.P., M.C. PATH. (Churchill).

RHEUMATIC DISEASES

Diseases of the Joints and Rheumatism by Kenneth Stone (Heinemann).
Disorders of the Locomotor System including the Rheumatic Diseases by E.
    Fletcher (Livingstone).
Rheumatism and Soft Tissue Injuries by J. Cyriax (Hamish Hamilton
    Medical Books).
Rheumatoid Arthritis—A Handbook for Patients, published by the Empire
    Rheumatism Council.
Textbook of the Rheumatic Diseases, edited by W. S. C. Copeman (Living-
    stone).
The Rheumatic Diseases by G. D. Kersley (Heinemann).
Textbook of Orthopaedic Medicine by J. Cyriax (Cassell).
Fracture and Joint Injuries by Sir Reginald Watson-Jones (Livingstone).

DISEASES OF THE RESPIRATORY SYSTEM

A Handbook of Chest Surgery for Nurses by J. Leigh Collis and L. E.
    Mabbit (Baillière, Tindall and Cassell).
The Anatomy of the Bronchial Tree by R. C. Brock (Oxford University
    Press).
Diseases of the Chest by R. Coope (Livingstone).
A Practice of Thoracic Surgery by A. L. d'Abreu (Edward Arnold).
Physiotherapy, Dec. 1966, 'Breathing Exercises in Emphysema' by D. M.
    Innocenti, M.C.S.P.

DISEASES OF THE NERVOUS SYSTEM

Diseases of the Nervous System by W. R. Brain (Oxford University Press).
Diseases of the Nervous System by F. N. R. Walshe (Livingstone).
Introduction to Clinical Neurology by Gordon Holmes (Livingstone).
Peripheral Nerve Injuries by Haymaker and Woodhall (W. B. Saunders).
Poliomyelitis by W. Ritchie Russell (Edward Arnold).
Muscle Testing and Function by Henry O. Kendall and Florence P. Kendall (The Williams and Wilkins Company).
Orthopaedic Surgery by Walter Mercer (Edward Arnold).
Essentials of Orthopaedics by Philip Wiles (Churchill).
Outline of Orthopaedics by John Crawford Adams (Livingstone).
Cerebral Palsy in Childhood and Adolescence: A Medical, Psychological and Social Study, edited by J. L. Henderson (Livingstone).
'Physical Methods Used in the Diagnosis and Treatment of Neuro-Muscular Disorders' by R. E. M. Bowden in *Physical Medicine and Rehabilitation*, edited by B. Kiernander (Blackwell).
Physiotherapy in Paraplegia by Elvira Hobson, F.C.S.P. (Churchill).

DISEASES OF THE SKIN

Common Skin Diseases by A. C. Roxburgh, revised by P. Borrie (Lewis).
Gardiner's Handbook of Skin Diseases, revised by John Kinnear (Livingstone).
Diseases of the Skin by John T. Ingram and Reginald T. Brain (Churchill).
Nursing and Management of Skin Diseases by D. S. Wilkinson (Faber and Faber).

MANAGEMENT OF PHYSICAL DISABILITY

Social Services in Britain, H.M.S.O., 1966.
Public Social Services (12th edition), National Council of Social Service 1965.
Voluntary Social Services, National Council of Social Service 1965, Supplement 1967.
The Social Services of Modern England by M. Penelope Hall (Routledge & Kegan Paul, 1965).
Designing for the Disabled by Selwyn Goldsmith, Technical Information Service of the Royal Institute of British Architects.
Equipment for the Disabled (4 volumes), National Fund for Research into Crippling Diseases.

Welfare Services for the Physically Handicapped, Central Council for the Disabled.

Rehabilitation and Care of the Disabled in Britain, Reference Division, Central Office of Information.

Services for the Disabled, H.M.S.O., 1961.

Help for the Handicapped, National Council of Social Service.

Conveyance of the disabled, Spastics Society for the Joint Committee on Mobility for the Disabled.

List of Special Schools for Handicapped Pupils in England & Wales, Department of Education and Science, H.M.S.O., 1969.

Holidays for the Physically Handicapped, jointly, by Central Council for the Disabled and the British Red Cross Society.

Personal care of the elderly, Report of 14th National Conference on Care of the Elderly, N.C.S.S., 1968.

The Elderly, Handbook on Care and Services, National Council of Social Service, 1968.

Looking after old people at home by Doreen Norton, National Council of Social Service for National Old Peoples Welfare Council, 1962.

Index